THE *Promise* OF

hCG

How to banish fat, resculpt your body & rebalance your metabolism

Dr. Sherrill Sellman, ND
Frankie Boyer

LEGAL DISCLAIMER:

The FDA has not approved hCG Therapy to lose weight.

"hCG has not been demonstrated to be effective adjunctive therapy in the treatment of obesity. There is no substantial evidence that it increases weight loss beyond that resulting from caloric restriction, that it causes a more attractive or "normal" distribution of fat, or that it decreases the hunger and discomfort associated with calorie-restricted diets."

ISBN: 978-0-9844733-3-5

Published By:

Bridger House Publishers, Inc.
PO Box 599, Hayden ID, 83835
1-800-729-4131

Cover Design & Typesetting: Julie Melton, The Right Type, USA
therighttype.com

Printed in the United States of America

10 9 8 7 6 5 4 3 2 1

Other Titles by
Dr. Sherrill Sellman, ND

Books

*Hormone Heresy: What Women MUST Know
About Their Hormones*

*What Women MUST Know To Protect Their Daughters
From Breast Cancer*

Salba: The Return of the Ancient Seed

Audio Programs

Getting Your Hormones Back On Track

DVD Programs

*What Women MUST Know to Protect Their Daughters
From Breast Cancer*

Table of Contents

Foreword

Dr. Sherrill's Story

Like so many women, the mid-life middle spread seemed to have sneaked up on me. I knew I had just emerged from two years of major life changes with its accompanying stress. Well, really, to be totally honest, MAJOR STRESS! However, I was not at all prepared for my doctor's rather blunt comment.

Rather tactlessly he said. "What has happened to you? You look like you are six months pregnant."

I knew I had been carrying some extra cortisol-induced weight around the midriff, but I guess denial is a really wonderful thing. I really didn't think I looked that overweight. Certainly not enough to look six months pregnant! Stepping onto his scale really ripped the veil of illusion from my eyes!

For most women, weight gain is the bane of our existence. Culturally, we all suffer from a fat phobia. Putting our vanity aside, extra-weight — just ten pounds — is a potential health hazard. In 2004 the U.S. Centers for Disease Control and Prevention (CDC) ranked obesity as the number one health threat facing America. More than 60 percent of women over the age of 20 fall into the overweight category. That makes it 64.5 million of us! And, if we're talking obesity that means almost 35 million more are in that category.

Americans spend a lot of money on weight loss programs and diets — $50 billion annually!

That's an awful lot of our hard earned cash! And here's the rub, within five years of losing weight, 95 percent of people will gain it all back and more!

Whether we like it or not, the older we get the less efficient our body becomes at detoxifying, maintaining a dynamic metabolism, balancing hormones and managing blood sugar. All of these issues can add to ever upward-creeping weight. Popular drugs also play their part. It is well acknowledged that HRT, anti-depressants, statins, and blood pressure medications list weight gain as side effects!

I have not been immune from this obsession with body image. There were times when I have been thin. And then there were times when I have been fat. I dieted and fasted and cleansed and starved and exercised until I was blue in the face!

Over the years I refined my nutritional regime. I basically ate a gluten-free, sugar-free, soda-free, processed-food free, organic food diet. I exercised (sometimes). I made the extra effort to manage my stress levels. I took my nutritional supplements. I balanced my hormones (naturally). I went to sleep at a decent hour (going to bed after 11pm and getting less than 7 hours can increase weight).

I thought I was doing everything right but my weight loss was stalled. I couldn't get it to budge. So, it's no wonder that my doctor's comment was such a blow to my self-image and my fruitless efforts!

One day, a chance comment about a new kind of weight loss program changed my life. I was introduced to hCG, Human Chorionic Gonatrophin, an obscure hormone that I had never heard of before.

It seems that hCG plays a major role in our survival. I learned that although it is produced in the bodies of men and women, it is found in very high amounts during pregnancy. One of its jobs is to ensure the survival of the pregnant mother and fetus by signaling the hypothalamus to release stored fat to be used as fuel and nourishment.

It is also called into action in times of starvation. Under the command of hCG, these fat reserves will provide 1,500-4,000 calories a day of energy and nutrition.

However, it is important to emphasize that hCG is not a sex hormone. Its action is identical in men, women, and children, young and old alike.

What hCG does for a pregnant women, is what it can also do for us. This amazing hormone has become the key ingredient to one of the most successful permanent fat loss and resculpting programs ever created. We have Dr. A.T.W. Simeons to thank for that.

Dr. Simeons was a brilliant English medical doctor who discovered that hCG had a major impact on fat loss by regulating the hypothalamus. The main function of this master gland is homeostasis, or maintaining the body's status quo. Ultimately the hypothalamus can control every endocrine gland in the body. It also regulates other factors such as blood pressure, body temperature, fluid and electrolyte balance, and body weight.

The message that hCG gives the body is to release reserves of long-term stored fat. That's the ugly fat that we struggle so hard to rid ourselves of. It's the fat that is stored in our abdomen, thighs and hips. That is also the fat that accumulates as fat pads in our arms, knees, back and neck. The most frustrating thing about this variety of fat is that no amount of dieting will ever touch it. It is only accessible with hCG. The body seems to hold on to it for dear life as part of its survival strategy.

The first to go when we start dieting is water, muscle and subcutaneous fat — the fat that gives shape to our face and fullness to our breasts. No wonder most diets result in saggy and toneless skin.

But hCG is totally different. It releases ONLY the long-term stored fat, it actually helps the body to properly redistribute weight and regain firmness in the body. So on the hCG program you not only lose pounds, you lose inches! No sagging...no loose skin. In fact, it actually helps to tone your body.

And the most amazing thing is that Dr. Simeons' program allowed people to lose a pound of fat a day, on average. While most weight loss programs consider the loss of one or two pounds a week a great success, the hCG program enables people to lose as much as a pound a day...not to mention the melting of inches!

The real bonus of this program is the rebalancing of the body's metabolism. When the program is followed precisely, you are able to regain a healthy metabolism. This is key to making sure your weight will stay off. Yo-yoing can then become a thing of the past.

While Dr. Simeons' original program revolved around injections of hCG, there is now a more convenient and easy method to get the exact same results.

The body is literally able to read the information and create the desired outcome. In the case of homeopathic hCG, it has the exact same effect as the more unpleasant and expensive hCG hormone injections.

What really made me gun shy was learning that I had to do a daily subcutaneous injections of hCG. There was no way I would do that.

But I then learned that there was another hCG option. This involved taking sublingual drops of an hCG homeopathic remedy daily. Homeopathy, a 200-year-old healing approach, based on the emerging science of energy medicine that imprints the energy of a substance without using the actually physical substance.

To say I was skeptical would be an understatement. But, nothing ventured, nothing gained. And I was assured that the homeopathic drops were absolutely safe.

So, I decided to give it a try. Using the hCG homeopathic drops along with following Dr. Simeons' protocol of specific foods in specific amounts for a specific period of time I embarked on this experiment. The best part of all, this program requires no specific exercise routines nor expensive eating plans nor special dietary formulas.

Now for most of us, stepping onto a scale to weigh in is equivalent to engaging in an extreme masochistic act. However, on this hCG program, it was closer to a religious experience. I would step on the scale in the morning and literally discover that a pound of fat had literally dematerialized from my body every day.

But it wasn't only the pounds. It was also the inches. My old clothes were literally falling off me. I wasn't hungry at all. My energy was off the charts. And before my very eyes I saw my body transforming. The midriff disappeared and my hips and thighs have morphed into the reincarnation of my thin 16-year-old shape! An accomplishment I never thought possible in this lifetime! And wonders of wonders — my muscle tone actually improved.

Unbelievable!

During this 23-day protocol, I lost 15 pounds and 2 dress sizes!

I then followed this round with a second go. I transformed a bulging 168 pound, size 12 body into 140 pounds of svelte, easily donning a pair of size 6 jeans. I thought I had died and gone to heaven!

The most impressive part of this amazing program was that by resetting my hypothalamus and my metabolism, my weight has not varied more than a couple of pounds... and that was two years ago. It appears that Dr. Simeons was right. By improving metabolic functioning on the hCG program, there is a greater likelihood that this new weight loss is here to stay.

Since venturing into the hCG world, I have assisted over 500 of my patients and friends on this protocol. Every single one of them has been successful. Men seem to have a fat loss advantage over women; they are much bigger losers on this program. However, the good news is that everyone can be a big loser!

Beyond the pound and inches, there are tremendous health gains — joint and knee aches disappear, blood sugar and blood pressure level normalize, sleep improves, energy increases, skin tone rejuvenates and food cravings disappear.

It's not often that a weight loss program can deliver such fabulous results. In fact, there is no weight loss program that I know of that even comes close. The hCG protocol is an entirely new paradigm for transforming an overweight body.

Could the wonderful discovery of Dr. Simeons be the solution for the growing epidemic of the obesity epidemic with all of the accompanying chronic health problems?

I have no doubt that in our diet-crazed world of people desperately seeking help; this is truly is the ultimate fat loss and resculpting program!

Thank you, Dr. Simeons, for this answer to our prayers.

Frankie's Story

Frustration was a word that I knew only too well. As the host of my own radio show talking about holistic health every day, why, oh why, could I not lose weight? I really did eat healthy foods, so what was blocking me from losing weight? Did I burn out my adrenals and my thyroid? My good friend, Dr. Sherrill Sellman, shared some insight on the homeopathic product called hCG. My world began to change inch by inch.

A few years ago I went through a very difficult phase in my personal life. I was under tremendous pressures and, on top of all of the personal challenges, my beloved Black Chow Chow, Tu Tu, got sick. A week later she died at 13½ years old.

I began to notice that during these difficult days and nights my body was changing. I was gaining weight. How was this possible? I was getting up at 4:45am, 3 days a week and working out in a small group with a very intense trainer. After lamenting to Dr. Sellman about my frustrations of what can I possibly be doing wrong? I'm exercising like crazy, eating healthy organic foods and still losing this weight battle.

It was at that point that I decided to try the homeopathic version of the hCG protocol.

Phase one, the loading phase, included eating fats and foods that I had not eaten in decades. Currently my personal Phase 1 is a gluten and sugar free loading.

Within days of the Very Low Calorie Phase 2, I noticed the inches beginning to drop from my body. Not the pounds but the inches. I could see a real difference, my shape was changing.

As a vegetarian I had many doubts that this protocol would work for me. My weight loss did take a little bit longer than non-vegetarians but I began to see extraordinary differences. Within a few weeks, for the first time in years, I noticed my body looking thinner without exercising. My trainer did not approve of what I was doing. I decided to take a break from my intense workouts because I felt my body needed a rest.

I did a few rounds of the hCG protocol and was realizing that many, many changes were occurring. Not only was my body being transformed but I began to feel a total change inside and out. For me it was a real spiritual awakening. People stopped me and asked what I had been doing to myself to have such a glow. Now my lifestyle reflected how I felt *and* how I looked.

The fatty bags under my eyes were gone and so was the bloating I always had in my stomach. It was during this transformation that I realized how sensitive I had become to gluten. If it were not for the hCG protocol I never would have understood what life is like without gluten and all the wonderful foods I have created without sugar and gluten. I discovered an entire world of nutrient dense delicious foods.

I am thrilled with the results; it just continues to amaze me years later. There is 34 pounds less of me with over 30 inches gone. I am still glowing. This protocol has given me so much hope. I am feeling fit, shapely and sexy in size 6 jeans. I no longer wake up each day looking to hide my weight, looking for big clothes and feeling badly that I ate right and worked out but didn't look like I did.

For a detox that boosts self esteem, food cravings and makes you look years younger, hCG is the answer. As I say to all of my listeners, "Give me 23 days and I promise it will transform your life." I know it will work for you as well. If you are sick and tired and want to change your weight roller coaster, this protocol is the answer. And the best part is that the results are fast.

I say on air all of the time, "When you cross Mass Avenue outside Harvard Square at 117 pounds, they will stop short for you. When you cross that same street at 200 pounds, they will run you over." I have struggled with my weight for years but now I feel I have the solution and it is hCG.

Introduction:

Is the End of Obesity in Sight?

Thank you Dr. Sherrill Sellman and Frankie Boyer for introducing me to this incredible program. Dr. Sellman and a growing number of doctors who are incorporating hCG programs into their clinical practices have all reported significant weight loss and successful maintenance.

I met Karen in 1963 when she was 16-years-old. We married in 1968. Forward ahead, 42 years of a wonderful marriage, 6 children, 10 grandchildren and 200+ additional pounds between us. My wife and I tried virtually every weight loss program that came on the market such as: liquid protein, powder protein, meal replacements, Atkins and countless others, even if they admitted the advertised results were atypical. All had limited weight loss success, zero long term success and often a weight gain afterwards. Why, like so many other people who have been successful in so many aspects of their lives, were we not able to control our weight? Why, like so many others, did we continue to gain weight and be severely overweight?

I had been reading about a program by the late Dr. Simeons which consisted of low dose, hCG (Human Chorionic Gonadatropin) along with a VLCD (very low calorie diet) which had enormous success in his patients for the treatment of obesity and Metabolic Syndrome. He explained his theory and documented his findings in his manuscript entitled *Pounds and Inches.* Metabolic Syndrome consists of some or all of the following: elevated blood pressure, elevated cholesterol, elevated triglycerides, insulin resistance and central obesity. Dr. Simeons purported that his hCG protocol would cause weight loss and reduce inches by mobilizing abnormal fat stores in the abdomen, neck, arms and legs. By doing so it would lower or eliminate the need for pharmaceuticals to treat the symptoms of Metabolic Syndrome.

In September 2009 I was a guest speaker at the A4M (American Academy of Anti-Aging Physicians) Conference in San Jose. The A4M Conference brings together physicians, pharmacists, and other health care practitioners who practice anti-aging and rejuvenative medicine. Over the five years that I have been a speaker there I have met many professionals who treat Metabolic Syndrome and obesity. At the Conference I spoke with pharmacists and physicians who utilize the hCG programs in their clinical practices. Some of the pharmacists were able to compound hCG into a low dose sublingual solution negating the need for daily injections. I was also inspired by a medical school classmate of mine who used the Dr. Simeons' hCG program in 2004, lost more than 70 pounds and not regained any of the weight in over five years.

This convergence of events led me, in September 2009, at the age of 63, 6' tall and weighing 334 pounds, to start the hCG program, using the prescription pharmaceutical sublingual hCG that was prepared by one of the compounding pharmacists at the Conference. At the same time, my oldest son Jeremy (6'1" - 275 pounds), an attorney, joined me. After one month I had lost almost 30 pounds and Jeremy lost approximately 25 pounds. In October my wife, Karen, (5'4½," - 230 pounds) and my daughter, Jennifer, (5'7," - 225 pounds), an Associate Professor of Nursing at DePaul University, joined us.

By Christmas 2009, I was down to 275 pounds, the lowest weight I had been in more than 30 years. For the first time in over 30 years I had normal blood pressure readings, no longer needing prescription pharmaceuticals to control it. For the first time in many years the weight on my driver's license was more than my actual weight.

I integrated the hCG program into my practice in March 2010. I had a dual purpose for doing this as I would be the inspiration for my patients and they would be mine. To date we have had approximately 500 patients, more than 400 have stayed with the program and have collectively lost over 9 TONS! Many of the patients have reduced their need for prescription pharmaceuticals for controlling blood pressure, cholesterol and blood sugar and others have eliminated the need completely as their metabolic values have become normal. Just today (January 17, 2011) I received an email from one of my patients, who has joined me in the 100 pound weight loss club. He is the sixth patient of mine to join this elite club — an incredible achievement. We have had more than 100 patients who have lost more than 50 pounds and many who have lost between 20 and 50 pounds (not everyone needs to lose as much weight as I did). To date my wife and daughter have lost over 70 pounds each, my son, over 50 pounds, and myself over 100 pounds.

I am so grateful to Dr. Sellman, A4M and the other medical professionals who are making this hCG protocol available. They have helped me accomplish, in a relatively short period of time, something which I never thought was possible. Thank you, thank you, thank you.

****

Dr. Mayer Eisenstein, MD, JD, MPH, is a graduate of the University of Illinois Medical School, the Medical College of Wisconsin School of Public Health, and the John Marshall Law School. In his 38 years in medicine, he and his practice have cared for over 75,000, children, parents, and grandparents. He is the founder and Medical Director of the Homefirst® Health

Services. He is Board Certified by the American Board of Public Health and Preventive Medicine, and the American Board of Quality Assurance and Utilization Review Physicians. He is a member of the Illinois Bar.

His latest book, *Making An Informed Vaccine Decision* goes along with his other books: *Give Birth at Home With The Home Birth Advantage; Safer Medicine, Don't Vaccinate Before You Educate, 2nd Edition; Unavoidably Dangerous – Medical Hazards of HRT* and *Unlocking Nature's Pharmacy.* Some of his many guest appearances include: "The Oprah Winfrey Show" and "Hannity and Colmes." His weekly syndicated radio show, "The Dr. Mayer Eisenstein Show," airs in the Chicagoland area. One of his goals is to lower the use of pharmaceuticals in the American population.

Chapter 1

An Effective Solution to the Obesity Epidemic

Look around.

Notice anything?

Our world is getting fatter… much fatter. Never before in the history of humanity have such corpulent bodies walked the earth.

Now that the average American is carrying around 23 extra pounds of fat, we are becoming a super-sized country. And, there is no way to disguise the transformation occurring in bodies of both young and old.

The reality of the growing girth of Americans and the ensuing 30 or more health conditions associated with this extra fat is putting America on a fast track to a national health disaster.

According to government data, about 66 percent of people are now either overweight or obese, which is defined as 30 or more pounds over a healthy weight.

However, the weight categories keep expanding. There are more than 3 million Americans who really topple the scales as morbidly obese which means they are more than 100 pounds over their ideal weight and have a Body Mass (BMI) of greater than 40. (The BMI is a measurement of the relative percentages of fat and muscle mass in the human body, which is used as an index of obesity.)

And there is even more. People are getting so fat that new categories have been created to accurately define the growing fatness of people. Once the term "morbidly obese" described a small segment of the population, but beyond this is now the "super-obese" category. The super-obese have a body mass index of 50 or more and weigh upwards of 440 pounds. It is predicted that the ranks of the super-obese will double in the next decade.

It's mind boggling to comprehend what these statistics are revealing. Our overweightedness as a national trend is a grow-ing problem, figuratively and literally. According to the latest government statistics, the number of obese American adults outweighs the number of those who are merely overweight. The National Center for Health Statistics shows that more than 34 percent of Americans are obese, compared to 32.7 percent who are overweight. A little under 6 percent are "extremely" obese.

That translates into more than one-third of adults, or over 72 million people were obese in 2005-2006.

By the time 2030 rolls around, over 86 percent of American adults will be overweight or obese.[1]

Children are following the lead of their parents. The percentage of overweight children in the United States is growing at an alarming rate, with 1 out of 3 kids now considered overweight or obese. Approximately nine million children over six years of age are considered obese. Obese children and adolescents are more likely to add to the ranks of obese adults.[2] For example, one study found that approximately 80 percent of children who were overweight at aged 10-15 years were obese adults by the age of 25.[3] It also found that if overweight begins before eight years of age, obesity in adulthood is likely to be more severe.

Even a Little is Too Much

Even if you do not fall into the overweight category, as few as 10 pounds above your ideal weight is heading you into the danger zone. Dr. Daniel O. Belluscio, internationally recognized obesity expert and director of the hCG research center, Buenos Aires, Argentina, warns: "Every disease has a beginning. Those 10 pounds that someone cannot seem to lose can also be seen as the beginning of a progressive disorder called obesity. This initial stage may last a number of years. Although the disease is not mature and the body may not be noticeably distorted, the dangers are clear."

As the body ages and metabolism slows down, the pounds can naturally pack on. "People who are 10 pounds too heavy now may be 35 pounds overweight within a decade," Belluscio warns. "Even at 10 pounds overweight, people are gambling with their health. Those 10 pounds signal the potential onset of hypertension, coronary artery disease, diabetes, osteoarthritis, and cancer — all the increased risk factors that come with obesity."

Up until recently, it was thought that a little extra padding might make us less aesthetically unappealing, but that was about the extent of it. Few people ever equated it as deadly health risk. Now we know the truth. We are carrying around a ticking tome bomb within us with just 10 extra pounds.

Our Overweighted World

What is happening in the U.S. is consistent with a global trend. Overweight and obese men, women and children now make up the majority of the population of most westernized countries. The USA (74.1 percent), Australia (67.4 percent), New Zealand (68.4 percent) and the UK (61 percent), have the distinction of being ranked as the top 25 most overweight countries in the world.

The World Health Organization (WHO) now describes the prevalence of obesity as an epidemic. (Obesity is defined by percentage of body fat. Women with more than 32 percent of their weight from fat and men with more than 25 percent are deemed obese.)

People all over the world are getting fatter than ever. Once considered a problem only in high-income countries, obesity is dramatically on the rise in low- and middle-income countries. As of recent years, there has been a growing recognition of an emerging epidemic of obesity in the developing societies. In fact, the rate of increase in obesity prevalence in developing countries can often exceed that in the industrialized world. Indeed, the yearly rate of increase in overweight and obesity in regions of Asia, Africa and South America is two- to fivefold that seen in the United States.

Some of the statistics revealing the impact of this epidemic are staggering:

- One in 10 British children is likely to become obese by 2015.[4]

- In New Zealand, a 2006–07 health survey found that one in three adults were overweight (36.3 percent) and one in four were obese (26.5 percent).[5]

- By 2025 the number of obese Australians will surpass those of healthy weight.

- In China, the proportion of obesity among children under the age of 15 increased from 15 percent in 1982 to 27 percent in 2004.

- Two in every three South Africans have a weight problem.

- In Egypt more than 25 percent of 4-year-olds are fat.[6]

- Excess weight has reached epidemic proportions globally, with more than one billion adults being either overweight or obese.[7]

- The WHO predicts there will be 2.3 billion overweight adults in the world by 2015, and more than 700 million of them will be obese.[8]

This current health crisis has created a growing panic around the world, threatening not only to overwhelm health care systems but also to create excessive financial burdens on governments. For example, the health cost of obesity in the U.S. is as high as US $147 billion annually, based on a new study from RTI International and the Centers for Disease Control and Prevention.[9] According to the latest research published in *The Medical Journal of Australia,* the total direct cost of overweight and obesity in Australia is $21 billion a year, double the previous estimates.[10]

By far the greatest cost of obesity is its serious threat to long-term health. Obesity is associated with more than 30 medical conditions including: diabetes, high blood pressure, high cholesterol and triglycerides, coronary artery disease (CAD), strokes, gallbladder disease and cancers of the breast, prostate and colon. The non-fatal but debilitating health problems associated with obesity include respiratory difficulties, chronic musculoskeletal problems, varicose veins, skin problems, osteoarthritis, Alzheimer's Disease, gout, sleep apnea, infertility and psychological disorders. Obesity puts more stress on joints causing them to wear out prematurely. This helps to explain why the majority of joint and hip replacements involve overweight people.

And then there is the toll to one's self-esteem and self-image, which is immeasurable. No wonder that depression and anxiety are more common in overweight people.

While the costs to health and to government coffers are enormous, there is a booming business to be made out of this health disaster. The profits of the weight loss industry are overflowing. Americans spend over $59 billion a year on weight loss programs. In 2006, Weight Watchers' products and services alone netted $3 billion worldwide.[11]

In an effort to find a solution to this problem, the latest trend is the growing popularity of bariatric weight reduction operations like gastric banding, gastric bypass and variants of these stomach surgeries. Demand for weight loss surgery is soaring, with more than 100,000 procedures performed annually. It is estimated that over the next few years the total number of obesity surgery patients in the United States will exceed one million. The average cost is $30,000 per procedure. According to a University of Washington study, as many as one in 50 people die within one month of having gastric bypass surgery, and that figure jumps nearly fivefold if the surgeon is inexperienced.[12]

What's Really Going On?

Obesity is a modern problem. Statistics about it did not even exist 50 years ago. Yet, in just several decades the growing corpulence of millions of people threatens not only their health but also the health of future generations. Fingers point at the "obesogenic" nature of western diets and lifestyles that promote the increased intake of refined, high-carbohydrate, high-sugar-ladened and nutrient-depleted foods as well as physical inactivity.

Obviously, something is seriously amiss. Our bodies, especially our metabolism, seem to be going haywire. The paradox of this overweight condition is that some people are getting fatter, even though they're eating fewer calories and exercising more. Healthier dietary and lifestyle choices don't seem to be effective in shedding excess pounds. The tried and true strategy of the past: reducing calories and increasing exercise, is ineffective for the modern day battle of the bulge. The bulge just doesn't seem to want to budge.

So, what is the problem?

If we are truly seeking a solution to obesity, we need to look elsewhere. Traditional weight loss theories and dietary and lifestyle approaches are falling far short of stemming the tide. Societies are drowning in fat.

An organization such as Weight Watchers considers the loss of one to two pounds a week, a rousing success. That's a long, slow and demoralizing path to any significant weight loss. It's a challenge just to keep up one's enthusiasm for the long haul much less actually attain any significant weight loss. Try as hard as most people will on their latest diet plan; the odds are against them for any real success.

And then there is the issue of keeping it off. That's another huge hurdle.

So, what is really going on here? Are LAP-BANDs the future many of us will have to look forward to?

If we are going to find a truly effective answer to this health crisis, it's obvious we will have to look "outside the box" for the answers.

And that is exactly where one very determined doctor looked — "outside the box."

Chapter 2

A New Paradigm for an Obesity Epidemic Solution

As the weight on the scales in our collective corpulence continues to keep inching ever upwards, it's obvious that the traditional weight loss approach no longer works. In the past, the old dieting trick of reducing our caloric load and adding some aerobic exercise would do the job. "Calories in" were cut down and "calories out" were revved up. So, as people ate their salads and ran a marathon on their treadmills, the dream of a slimmer, leaner body consoled them. These days no amount of grazing on spring greens or dedication to the hours of running in place can budge the scale in a downward direction in any significant way. So many people have resigned themselves to a lifetime of being overweight.

What was a perfect weight loss formula in the past, fails us dismally in the present.

An unlikely hero would change all that.

A brilliant British endocrinologist, Dr. A.T.W. Simeons discovered a revolutionary approach to weight loss. Dr. Simeons graduated Summa Cum Laude in medicine from the University of Heidelberg. He spent many years working in India working with the government of India where he conducted extensive research on bubonic plague and leprosy control. In 1931 he was awarded the Red Cross Order of Merit by the Queen of England for his injection remedy for malaria and a method of staining malarial parasites, which is known as "Simeons' Stain."

In 1949, with his wife and three sons, he moved to Rome, where he worked on psychosomatic disorders at the Salvator Mundi International Hospital. While in Rome, he became fascinated with the problem of obesity and decided to set his brilliant mind on the task of researching its cause and its solution.

Little did he know that this search would be come his life's mission. He committed more than 20 years of his life to seeking the answer to the underlying cause of obesity and, then, establishing a clinic based upon his successful protocol. His reputation for a safe and effective weight loss program spread far and wide. Celebrities, movie stars and royalty from all over the world were treated at this clinic. Word of his success also led to other clinics throughout Europe incorporating the Simeons' protocol. Many exist to this day and continue to offer his program.

His research led him to investigate the links between endocrinology, obesity and psychosomatic disorders. He studied every potential solution for obesity offered anywhere in the world. One by one, he eliminated the potential underlying cause of the problem: the thyroid, pituitary, adrenal glands, pancreas, gallbladder and over 100 other physiological functions. He could find no direct correlation between obesity and these various glands and organs. The usual suspects were innocent.

He was sure that there was an unrecognized mechanism at work that was driving the obesity epidemic. It took decades before all the pieces of the puzzle would come together for him.

In his book, *Pounds and Inches: A New Approach to Obesity,*
Dr. Simeons recounts:

> What I have to say is an essence of views distilled out of
> forty years of grappling with the fundamental problems
> of obesity, its causes, its symptoms, and its very nature.
> In these many years of specialized work, thousands of
> cases have passed through my hands and were care-
> fully studied. Every new theory, every new method,
> every promising lead was considered, experimentally
> screened and critically evaluated as soon as it became
> known. But invariably the results were disappointing
> and lacking in uniformity. I felt that we were merely
> nibbling at the fringe of a great problem, as, indeed, do
> most serious students of overweight. We have grown
> pretty sure that the tendency to accumulate abnormal
> fat is a very definite metabolic disorder, much as is, for
> instance, diabetes.
>
> Yet the localization and the nature of this disorder re-
> mained a mystery. Every new approach seemed to lead
> into a blind alley, and though patients were told that they
> are fat because they eat too much, we believed that this is
> neither the whole truth nor the last word in the matter.
>
> Refusing to be side-tracked by an all too facile interpre-
> tation of obesity, I have always held that overeating is
> the result of the disorder, not its cause, and that "we can
> make little headway until we can build for ourselves
> some sort of theoretical structure with which to explain
> the condition. Whether such a structure represents the
> truth is not important at this moment. What it must do
> is to give us an intellectually satisfying interpretation of
> what is happening in the obese body. It must also be able
> to withstand the onslaught of all hitherto known clinical
> facts and furnish a hard background against which the
> results of treatment can be accurately assessed.

His determination finally paid off. He arrived at a major discovery. Dr. Simeons came to the conclusion that the underlying cause of obesity was to be found within the part of the brain called the diencephalon, a complex of structures that includes the thalamus and hypothalamus. He discovered that the origin of the problem was the compromised function of the hypothalamus.

According to Dr. Simeons:

> If obesity is always due to one very specific diencephalic deficiency, it follows that the only way to cure it is to correct this deficiency. At first this seemed an utterly hopeless undertaking. The greatest obstacle was that one could hardly hope to correct an inherited trait localized deep inside the brain, and while we did possess a number of drugs whose point of action was believed to be in the diencephalon, none of them had the slightest effect on the fat center. There was not even a pointer showing a direction in which pharmacological research could move to find a drug that had such a specific action.[13]

While it was commonly believed that overeating caused obesity, Simeons found the opposite to be true, that overeating is the result of a metabolic disorder—not its cause.

Dr. Simeons formulated a new theory about obesity. He elaborated upon the following "maxims."

Maxim #1: Obesity is a disorder.

Disorders occur when an organ or other body part no longer functions normally. So obesity is the consequence of compromised functioning.

Maxim #2: Abnormal fat is always caused by obesity.

After gaining a limited amount of weight, your body automatically stops unless you have the obesity disorder. Large fat deposits don't begin to develop until you have the obesity disorder.

Maxim #3: Obesity is not caused by overeating. Rather, over-eating is caused by obesity.

Sudden, intense cravings strike at obese people because they have the obesity disorder, not because they are greedy. Such attacks of hunger aren't the same thing as compulsive eating — they aren't psychological. They're physical. It simply takes more energy to maintain an obese or overweight body. By experience, your body knows that sugar provides the most fuel in the shortest amount of time. Because of that, it sends signals generating a desire for sweets.

Maxim #4: If you suffer from obesity, you will get fat no matter how much you eat.

The reason you become obese is because of the malfunction in your body that causes obesity. Your fat deposits get fed and sealed away before anything else, thanks to the obesity disorder.

Maxim #5: Regardless of how much you eat, if you do not have the obesity disorder, you will not become overweight.

Some people can gorge themselves and still stay thin as can be. Aren't they just lucky? Over time, however, they may also find that metabolism will begin to slow down.

Following along this line of reasoning, Dr. Simeons sought a treatment aimed at curing the disorder. His solution had to achieve the following criteria: it needed to be effective for both women and men; it must be successful for all forms of obesity; it must actually correct the disorder; and people must be able to resume eating normally without gaining abnormal fat.

What a tall order!

In Search of a Solution

The first part of the puzzle was to uncover the cause. Dr. Simeons was convinced that a dysfunctional hypothalamus was the long-sought-after answer. Now he was in pursuit of the solution.

His observations as well as unique experiences while working as a medical doctor in India provided him with the critical clues he was seeking.

His "Eureka moment" came when he remembered observing very thin pregnant Indian women, who, although eating a low-caloric intake and at the same time doing demanding physical activity, delivered healthy full-weight babies. These pregnant women could easily lose weight by drastically reducing their dietary intake but without feeling hungry or in any way harming the child in the womb. After much research, he attributed this phenomenon to the presence of a hormone-like substance called human chorionic gonadotrophin (hCG), which is made in high amounts in a woman's body during pregnancy.

He also reflected upon an unusual syndrome he observed while in India. It was a rare medical condition (Frohlich's Syndrome, or adiposogenital dystrophy) found in young obese Indian boys, known as "fat boys." Daily injections of small amounts of hCG totally cured them of their obesity. They miraculously lost their ravenous appetites and reshaped their bodies to a normal weight.

Calling upon his experiences, while in India, Dr. Simeons wondered if hCG could assist in opening the abnormal, secure reserves of fat in non-pregnant women and possibly even in men. Under normal conditions, these abnormal fat reserves are almost impossible to access and are only released as the body's last survival strategy during times of extreme starvation.

However, Dr. Simeons found one very interesting exception: hCG signals the body to mobilize these fat reserves.

At his Rome hospital, he experimented with this approach: daily hCG injections combined with a very specific 500-calories-per-day diet. After many years of working with thousands of test patients, he perfected his "weight loss cure protocol." The results were astonishing. Almost 100 percent of his patients were losing approximately one pound (0.45 kilogram) per day while on the protocol. And they were only losing the most difficult and resistant form of body fat to release—abnormal stored fat.

Was hCG the key that could safely and successfully reset a dysregulated hypothalamus?

The Hypothalamus Gland: The Missing Piece of the Fat Puzzle

The answer was to be found deep within our brain.

The problem of fat storage, which results in being overweight and obese, seems to be related to the master gland, the hypothalamus. The hypothalamus is a collection of specialized cells located immediately below the thalamus at the center of the brain, allowing communication between the endocrine and central nervous systems.

The hypothalamus gland is the equivalent of the master switch of the body overseeing and commanding many key autonomic functions of the body. It is one of the central elements of the brain and comprises the neuronal circuitry that controls emotional behavior and motivational drives. Without proper hypothalamic function, the two systems fail to respond appropriately to each other's signals.

Very simply, the hypothalamus organizes and controls many complex emotions, feelings and moods, as well as all motivational states including; hunger, appetite and food intake, and everything to do with the concept of pleasure including satisfaction, comfort and creative activities.

It works in conjunction with your pituitary gland to control all of your hormones.

And, a proper functioning hypothalamus is vital to regulate efficient fat burning.

If this part of your brain falls out of balance—which happens in response to stress, trauma, toxins, electromagnetic fields, yoyo dieting, etc.—you can experience excessive hunger, impaired metabolism, and accumulation of abnormal fat in various parts of your body such as your abdomen, hips, thighs, upper arms, and waist.

Getting Up Close and Personal with Your Hypothalamus

The neurons in the hypothalamus produce a number of hypothalamic neurotransmitters, which relay information and instruction to all parts of the brain and body, directly influencing the pituitary gland, where growth hormone, thyroid hormone releasing factor and other neuropeptides are released via hypothalamic input.

The hypothalamus (with the cerebral hemispheres) is intimately involved in the integration of all physiological stimulation, all 5 senses, including taste, smell, sight, sound, and touch, which it then translates, distills and assembles into one discernible "package," relating all the attributes of an experience, all the associated stimulation into one clear harmonious concept, one memory, one experience. Thus, yielding a succinct emotionally satisfying understanding and judgment of the experience itself.

The hypothalamus gland also produces secretions that are important to the management of cardiovascular function, certain metabolic activities such as the delicate maintenance of water balance, sugar and fat metabolism, body temperature control, appropriate sleep programming, appetite and thirst responses. The secretion of all hormones is facilitated by the hypothalamus. It is also involved in control of the pituitary gland.

Hidden within the hypothalamus is a satiety center that regulates appetite. It is controlled by two chemicals that stimulate the surrounding hypothalamus to increase metabolism, reduce appetite and increase insulin to deliver energy to cells rather than to be stored as fat. Unfortunately, these systems can be easily compromised.

The endocrine system is an intricate "feedback" system in which hormones release or suppress other hormones, controlling the way the body works. Balance is crucial because an unhealthy gland could cause repercussions to cascade down into all parts of the body.

It appears that our 21st-century lifestyle is a serious threat to a healthy, well-functioning hypothalamus. An imbalance of the hypothalamus results in intense and constant hunger, low metabolism, and excessive and abnormal storing of fat in abnormal fat reserves known as problem, disfiguring areas in the abdomen, hips, thighs, waist and various fat pads placed around the body.

It is very important to note that this gland does not operate normally in people who are fat. In fact, even the mildly overweight may also have an impaired hypothalamus. So, just holding on to an extra ten pounds can be a symptom that your hypothalamus is in trouble.

The main function of the hypothalamus is homeostasis, or maintaining the body's status quo. Factors such as blood pressure, body temperature, fluid and electrolyte balance, and body weight are held to a precise value called the set point. Although this set point can migrate over time, from day to day it is remarkably fixed.

Understanding the Hypothalamus

The general functions of the hypothalamus are of extreme importance for the body, such as:

- bladder function
- blood pressure regulation
- body temperature regulation
- energy levels
- feeding reflexes
- heart rate
- hormonal/neurotransmitter regulation (serotonin, dopamine, norepinephrine and acetylcholine)
- hunger and salt cravings
- hydration
- metabolism
- mood and behavioral functions
- ovarian function
- pituitary gland regulation
- sleep cycles
- testicular function
- thirst
- wakefulness
- water preservation

What Happens When The Hypothalamus Doesn't Work Properly?

The hypothalamus is a very sensitive gland.

When the hypothalamus is not working correctly, when it's not functioning up to par, the wrong neuro-signals are generated and the wrong neuro-messages are received. This results in an inaccurate integration of all our sensory input, leading to faulty perceptions which are very subtle but nonetheless powerful. This makes us feel empty, deprived and emotionally "unsatisfied." Dysfunction of the hypothalamus often leads to depression, hyperactivity, abnormal responses to stress, or disturbances in brain and limbic functioning.

Some of the physical aspects of hypothalamic dysfunction include: disordered sleep, multiple hormonal dysfunctions, immune dysfunction, food cravings autonomic dysfunction, altered body temperatures.

One of the most important messages that suffers is the command to burn fat. When your hypothalamus is misbehaving, you will put on fat regardless of whether you eat excessively, normally or minimally, and no amount of dieting will cause your abnormal fat stores to budge.

Wayward Weight: Blame it on the Hypothalamus

It appears that almost everything the hypothalamus does is related in some way to proper weight management and controlled weight loss. When the hypothalamus is dysfunctional, food becomes increasingly more important, but at the same time, less fulfilling. We end up feeling unsatisfied with the foods, which we have eaten, gradually eating more and more to try to compensate for whatever is lacking! From a metabolism stand point, the hypothalamus not only governs the motivation to eat, stimulating hunger and appetite, but most importantly how the eating experience is perceived. Without a healthy hypothalamus, eating is no longer seems pleasurable nor satisfying.

We are exposed to many modern days that exert great stress on the hypothalamus. Many things can have a serious impact on its proper functioning. It is adversely affected by stress and trauma, cycles of fasting and bingeing, and a toxic diet of highly refined, low-fiber foods contaminated with tens of thousands of man-made chemicals and additives. If all those factors weren't challenging enough, the hypothalamic function becomes impaired with age. So as we grow older the hypothalamus becomes less and less responsive to giving and receiving the correct messages.

Prolonged stress releases a cascade of powerful stress chemicals that can affect the functioning of the hypothalamus. The stress can be emotional, physical or environmental. For example, studies have shown that induced stress from exposure to loud noises, such as traffic and airplane, can negatively impact the brain.

Cycles of dieting and overeating, a common behavior for people who attempt to lose weight, impact brain function. Research shows that after extended periods of excessive eating, brain connections are permanently altered on a molecular level.

When you add a diet based upon junk foods, hydrogenated oils, sugar, food additives, alcohol and tobacco, you have added another great insult to the brain's ability to function optimally.

Exposure to a toxic world is another affront to the sensitive hypothalamus. Many toxic chemicals are able to breach the blood-brain barrier and gain entry to the hypothalamus, where they cause serious disruption. For example, pervasive environmental estrogen disruptors such as nonylphenol and bisphenol-A have a direct adverse impact on the hypothalamus.

According to medical researcher Robert O. Becker, MD, electromagnetic fields (EMFs) also have upset the hypothalamus. "The sites of the greatest change—the brain's hypothalamus and cortex—were cause for concern. The hypothalamus, a nexus part of the brain for homeostasis, is a crucial link in the stress response. Any interference with cortical activity...would disrupt logical and associational thought..."[14]

In less than 30 years, almost 90 percent of the planet and its inhabitants have been engulfed by continuous exposure to unrelenting EMFs and wireless technologies. According to noted researcher Dr. Henry Lai: "The added stress of continual exposure to wireless frequencies from use of mobile phones and other wireless devices further challenges the brain."[15]

The 21st century has provided the perfect storm that pushes a healthy functioning hypothalamus over the edge. Perhaps our delicate brain, especially the major controlling center, the hypothalamus, has finally reached the tipping point from exposure to the many unrelenting toxic substances, physical and emotional stressors, and the ever-pervasive wireless technologies.

The plain, simple fact is that this gland does not operate normally in overweight people and probably is compromised to some degree in most people. In order to release stored fat reserves, increase metabolism and reduce unrelenting physical hunger, the hypothalamus must be rebalanced in both women and men.

Chapter 3

Not All Fat Is Equal

We don't think much about our fat. Fat is fat is fat to most of us. We usually think of it as a blubbery substance that we dream of getting suctioned out! However, there is much to fat that we never knew.

Dr. Simeons made some very important distinctions when it came to the different forms of fat that exist within our bodies. These distinctions are critical for real weight loss success.

He classified fat into three very different kinds: structural fat, normal or essential fat reserves and non-essential, abnormal stored fat.

Structural fat fills the gaps between various organs, a sort of packing material. That provides protection for the body's major organs and joints. It also performs such important functions as bedding the kidneys in soft elastic tissue, protecting the coronary arteries and keeping the skin smooth and taut. It gives contour to our face. In addition, it provides the springy cushion of fat under the bones of the feet enabling us to walk without pain.

Normal fat reserves are spread all over the body and are used for fuel when the body is faced with immediate nutritional or caloric insufficiencies. Fat is a substance that packs the highest caloric value into the smallest space so that normal reserves of fuel for muscular activity and the maintenance of body temperature can be most efficiently stored.

Both types of fats, structural and normal, are needed for good health. These types of fats will never contribute to obesity.

The third form of fat, however, is an entirely different story. Abnormal stored fat, or adipose fat, is kept in storage under the skin and around the organs as a "spare fuel supply" for severe nutritional emergencies. It is the accumulation of this kind of fat that results in being overweight or obese. In the obese person, it tends to collect in places like the abdomen, hips, buttocks, thighs, knees, ankles, upper arms and neck.

This abnormal fat is also a potential reserve of fuel, but unlike the normal reserves, it is not available to the body for nutritional reserves. It is, so to speak, locked away. Only under unusual circumstances, such as for the survival of the fetus or during times of severe starvation, will the body call upon it.

This is the fat that not only misshapes the body but also causes other serious adverse health consequences. Contrary to what most people think, abnormal fat is not simply an inert storehouse of unused calories encasing your body and organs. It is the most metabolically active tissue in the human body, nearly tripling the blood circulation of any other organ.

The abnormal fat also serves as an endocrine and secretory organ. Fat cells produce a bewildering array of biochemicals that influence what goes on in your body. One family of biochemicals produced by these abnormal fat cells is cytokines, many of which are involved in the inflammatory process. They include leptin, adiponectin, tumor necrosis factor alpha (TNF-alpha), interleukin-6 (IL-6), to name a few. Most cytokines promote inflammation while some others inhibit inflammation.

Abnormal fat cells increase inflammation in another way. They attract a type of white blood cell known as a macrophage, which also produces inflammatory cytokines. Macrophages are scavenger cells. Their job is literally to gobble up foreign organisms and cellular debris.

Macrophages seem to be drawn to abnormal fat because fat cells tend to leak and break open, especially in people with abdominal obesity. Macrophages move into the leaky fat tissue in order to clean up debris and then they themselves begin to release inflammatory factors. Macrophages appear to be a major contributor to inflammation.

The more abnormal fat cells you have, especially around your middle, the more cytokines you will produce and the more likely it is that you are promoting inflammation.

Fat cells are also little factories producing an enzyme called aromatase. This enzyme, in turn, makes a very potent form of estrogen, called estrone in both women and men. A vicious cycle is then initiated. Fat cells make estrone and estrone creates more fat cells. Estrone is also a pro-inflammatory hormone, adding to the dangerous inflammatory state occurring within an overweight or obese body.

Under normal dieting programs, the body will release structural and normal fat reserves. It will also burn muscle and water. The very last fat that a body will burn is abnormal fat reserves, since it is the body's final survival strategy for a severe malnourished body.

So, try as dieters might, all that bulging, distorting fat around the belly, hips and thighs will never be touched. Instead, they become gaunt, saggy and weak as they lose their structural and reserve fat supplies as well as muscle mass. This further diminishes hypothalamic functions.

The old dieting paradigm of eating less, exercising more and adding a few supplements into the mix is doomed to fail. That abnormal fat is locked away tight. The communication from the command center of the hypothalamus to the downstream glands and organs is scrambled. Directives are improperly interpreted. Functions are compromised.

It's this fact that makes the usual dieting strategies not only ineffective but actually exacerbate the very problem they are trying to solve.

The Three Types of Fat

Structural fat: This "good fat" protects your major organs and joints. It also provides contouring and sculpting of your face. It is ordinarily not burned for energy.

Normal fat reserves: Also "good fat," this type of fat is spread throughout your body to, ideally, be burned when your body needs immediate fuel. It's your regular gas tank.

Abnormal stored fat: Also called adipose fat, this type of fat is not needed and is what accumulates when a person becomes obese. It is stored underneath your skin and around your organs as a spare fuel supply, causing those unsightly bumps and bulges. It is metabolically active gland producing inflammatory chemicals and estrone. Your body accesses this as a final survival strategy should you become malnourished.

Chapter 4

hCG - The Key
That Releases the Fat

The true genius of Dr. Simeons was discovering the answer to the most fundamental questions. What would restore the functioning of a dysregulated hypothalamus? Was it possible to access the abnormal fat reserves and burn the fat? Could both women and men safely benefit? Would the results be permanent?

Dr. Simeons finally found the answer in the form of hormone-like substance called human chornionic gonadatrophin, or hCG. For most people, hCG is a new word that has been added to their hormone lexicon. Outside of the world of obstetrics most people have never heard of it before.

His revolutionary discovery was about to profoundly transform the bodies, health and lives of thousands upon thousands of people around the world.

A Word About hCG

Human chorionic gonadotropin (hCG) is the biggest glycoprotein, consisting of 244 amino acids present in human beings. It's not technically a hormone, although you will often hear it called one. This protein hormone is recognized as a peptide. Peptides are a class of hormone that is secreted into the blood stream and aide in endocrine functions in living animals.

hCG is important in triggering hormonal changes in women during pregnancy, embryo development and it can increase the production of natural male and female steroids (sex hormones).

It is a substance produced in huge amounts by the placenta during pregnancy. It almost completely controls the metabolic function through the hypothalamus throughout the pregnancy. Its role is to maintain the integrity of the corpus luteum of a pregnant woman's ovary in order to produce the hormone progesterone, which is essential to her growing fetus. In fact, hCG is actually what is being measured when you do a pregnancy test.

A pregnant woman makes between 500,000-1,000,000 IU. When injections of sublingual forms of hCG are used in the Simeons' protocol, they contain a very small amount of hCG, between 125-200 IU. The hCG used with injections or sublingually in the hCG diet protocol is a variation of the hCG form which is used for fertility treatments, but in a much smaller dose. All forms of the hCG hormone are created in a laboratory from sterile cells. It is NOT extracted from women or animal urine — a common misconception.

According to Daniel Belluscio, MD, Director of The Oral hCG Research Center in Buenos Aires, Argentina, "...hCG has been found in every human tissue, also in males and non-pregnant females. Investigators are very intrigued regarding the presence of hCG, for example in lungs, liver, stomach, etc."[16]

While Dr. Simeons pioneered the use of hCG in the form of injections, there are now other delivery options for the hCG program. It is possible to use the hormone in a sublingual form. Another alternative is the use of sublingual homeopathic hCG formulas. If used in conjunction with Dr. Simeons' precise dietary protocol, these various forms fulfill the promise of successfully melting away unwanted pounds and inches, safely and rapidly. And if Dr. Simeons' long-term program is followed, the changes are permanent.

Just to be clear, hCG is not the same thing as HGH—it's important to not confuse the two. HGH is human growth hormone, which also plays a major role in your metabolism. However, HGH is produced by your pituitary gland, particularly at night while you sleep, and in response to high-intensity, burst-type exercises that engage your super-fast muscle fibers.

hCG to the Rescue

Dr. Simeons discovered that hCG kept the structural fat and muscle intact while only breaking down the abnormal body fat, which was transformed into fuel by the body. The ability to release the stored toxic fat makes the fat reserves throughout the body readily accessible. In the presence of hCG, the body is able to transform the abnormal stored fat into what it was originally intended — 1,500-4,000 calories a day of energy and nutrition. The more stored fat a person had, the greater the daily fat loss would be.

People were amazed to find not only unwanted pounds disappearing on a daily basis, but their bodies were resculpting as inches disappeared from previously mis-shapened areas before their eyes!

Dr. Simeons' research revealed that hCG maximizes the functional capacity of all the centers in the hypothalamus, including what he termed the "fat center," making it possible for fat to be released from abnormal fat deposits and to become available as a source of fuel to the body.

This discovery led Dr. Simeons to write: "Someone suffering from obesity [who] attempts weight loss through a low-calorie diet will first lose lean muscle tissue, followed by protective visceral fat....only as a last resort will the body yield its abnormal reserves...by that time the patient usually feels so weak and hungry that the diet is abandoned."[17]

This is the tragedy of those who repeatedly attempt low-calorie diets that invariably fail.

> **Dr. Simeons concluded that when hCG is reintroduced into the adult body, it recalibrates the hypothalamus gland and helps unlock adipose deposits, making them available as a fuel source when calories are not otherwise available, as when eating a low-calorie diet. However, unlike the loss of lean muscle mass and structural fat from low-calorie diets, under the influence of hCG only the abnormal stored fat is released.**

Dr. Simeons developed a very specific protocol for the use of hCG along with a precise dietary plan. The program must be followed meticulously. People who need to lose 15 pounds (7 kilograms) or less require a 23-day protocol. And it can also be used for up to 40 days to lose 34 pounds (15 kilograms) at a time.

When hCG is given in conjunction with a very low caloric diet of 500 calories, a condition is simulated in the body, "tricking" it into acting as though it were dealing with an emergency starvation situation. As a result, the hypothalamus signals the release of stored fat reserves. Since about 1,500-4,000 calories of stored abnormal fat is transformed into energy and nutrition, there is a safe but rapid loss of fat, up to a pound or more a day (the more fat there is to lose, the more rapid the fat loss).

More remarkable is the rapid resculpting of the body as the abnormal and distorting fat reserves literally melt away, revealing a new contoured shape in the areas of the body that have been most resistant to change. The abdomen becomes flat, the hips and thighs return to normal proportions, and fat pads in the back, upper arms and knees disappear. At the same time, the body becomes more toned and the skin more radiant. As abnormal fat reserves are transformed into energy and nutrition, people report an abundance of energy and rarely, if ever, feel any hunger.

The best thing about hCG is that it is undeniably safe. Remember, pregnant women can experience high levels of hCG with no negative effects. The use of a small amount of the hormone, whether an injectable or sublingual form, during the weight loss program has very few side effects. The homeopathic hCG option, based upon the principles of homeopathy as an energy medicine, do not contain any of the actual hCG hormone in them at all.

The introduction of hCG is the key that makes Dr. Simeons' program a totally new paradigm for releasing stored fat. By using hCG with his low-calorie diet, extra fat is mobilized for energy. Following the dietary protocol precisely, which was created to accompany the use of hCG, is vital in preventing immediate refilling of emptied fat cells. You benefit by preferentially getting rid of excess fat without affecting bone and muscle.

Chapter 5

Restored Health with hCG

While the hCG protocol is extraordinary in its ability to facilitate the loss of the right kind of pounds and inches, the benefits don't stop there.

As the body releases and literally dissolves excess fat cells, people notice many health benefits. According to Dr. Simeons: "The most important associated disorders and the ones in which obesity seems to play a precipitating or at least an aggravating role are the following: diabetes, gout, rheumatism and arthritis, high blood pressure and hardening of the arteries, coronary disease and cerebral hemorrhage."

As the fat is transformed into energy, there is a reduction of chronic inflammation throughout the body. Since most health conditions and associated symptoms are caused by inflammation and the ensuing damage to tissues, people experience the resolution of a myriad of conditions and symptoms.

In addition, the hCG protocol vastly improves, if not totally resolves, the following: blood sugar and blood pressure return to normal range, moods and sleep improve, sugar and carbohydrate cravings disappear, triglyceride and cholesterol levels normalize. Aches and pains from arthritis disappear, as do many autoimmune conditions. Diabetes is reversed.

Since every extra pound translates into 4-5 pounds of additional pressure on the lower back, hips, knees, ankles and feet, pain reduces as the pounds disappear.

The hCG hormone generates endorphins in the human body, and these endorphins generate feelings of well being, increased energy and increase your ability to focus.

In addition, hCG rebalances the endocrine system. One aspect of the endocrine system that can improve is the thyroid. According to Dr. Simeons, contrary to popular belief, the thyroid plays no part in releasing the fat that causes us to be overweight.

> When it was discovered that the thyroid gland controls the rate at which body-fuel is consumed, it was thought that by administering thyroid gland to obese patients their abnormal fat deposits could be burned up more rapidly. This, too, proved to be entirely disappointing because, as we now know, these abnormal deposits take no part in the body's energy turnover—they are inaccessibly locked away. Thyroid medication merely forces the body to consume its normal fat reserves, which are already depleted in obese patients, and then to break down structurally essential fat without touching the abnormal deposits. In this way a patient may be brought to the brink of starvation in spite of having a hundred pounds of fat to spare. Thus any weight loss brought about by thyroid medication is always at the expense of fat of which the body is in dire need.

There seems to be great truth to Dr. Simeons' insights about the role of the thyroid in fat loss. Many people who are prescribed thyroid medication experience no significant weight loss at all. On the other hand, those who have committed to the hCG program have reported noticeably improvement in the functioning of their thyroid. The hCG protocol has assisted some people to eliminate the need for thyroid medication entirely. For others, their thyroid responded enough so that their medical practitioner was able to reduce their dose. However, this is not true for everyone. Whether you continue taking your thyroid medication while on the program, or discover you no longer have a need for it, the program will work either way.

Some Health Conditions Benefited with hCG:

1. Reduction in fasting blood sugar for type 2 diabetics

2. Reduction in aches and pains of various origin, including arthritis, and joint improvement

3. Reduced triglyceride and cholesterol levels

4. Reduction in blood pressure in those whose blood pressure was elevated

5. Reduced sugar and carbohydrate cravings

6. Balanced endocrine system, thyroid function improved

7. Improved Psoriasis, eczema, other skin conditions and varicose ulcers

8. Reduced levels of inflammation

In addition to the improvement or even resolution of more chronic health issues, people have reported many additional benefits. The combination of reducing the toxic, inflammatory load of abnormal fat reserves and the simple, cleansing diet that is a necessary pre-requisite of a successful program have amazed people with the many changes they experienced.

- Increased energy and vitality without hunger

- An end to food cravings

- Better skin tone

- Improved body shape and weight loss from problem areas

- Restoration of better hormonal balance

- A decrease or disappearance of hot flushes and period problems

- An end to ravenous hunger

- A beautifully sculpted body

- Deeper sleep

- Normalized appetite

- A new fat set point

- Greater self esteem

- An end to carbohydrate and sugar addictions

- Emotional balance

Chapter 6

The hCG Program is Head and Shoulders Above the Rest

It cannot be overstated that this program is worlds apart from any other weight loss program. While many programs attempt to correct the factors that impact the burning of calories, and hopefully some of the fat reserves, no other weight loss approach targets the primary cause of obesity. Only Dr. Simeons' hCG protocol has been demonstrated to correct a faulty hypothalamus. In fact, most other dieting regimes, will, in the end, only contribute to a slower and less efficient metabolism.

It is no surprise then why 95 to 98 percent of dieters regain the weight within one to five years. Doing the same old thing and expecting the outcomes to be different is delusional.

The hCG protocol has proven to literally rebalance the hypothalamus. It's as though the sensitive hypothalamus is rebooted back into action. Instead of having a less responsive metabolism, the body actually works much more efficiently. People are able to keep the weight off. The desire to eat is diminished and energy levels remain high.

This program also jump-starts people into a whole new way of relating to food and healthy life style choices. Imagine what is possible when you are free from carbohydrate and sugar cravings? And if you want motivation, try stepping on the scale every morning to discover another pound, more or less, has just disappeared.

The most powerful healing is to be able to stand in front of your mirror and see a thinner, toned, resculpted body reflected back at you. Self-loathing is transformed into self-love. Now that's really an answer to your prayers!

Consistent Results with hCG

Dr. Simeons published his research in the prestigious medical journal The Lancet in 1954. As a result of his stellar reputation, his meticulous research and outstanding results on thousands of patients, medical doctors around the world flocked to his technique. Exclusive clinics that catered to the rich and famous were established throughout Europe, and are still in existence today.

Yet, fearful of ridicule or more nefarious agendas from multinational corporations and the medical orthodoxy that were not favorable to a safe fat-loss cure, Dr. Simeons was most protective and secretive of his protocol. While there have been detractors to Dr. Simeons' work, some studies that have seemingly proven his protocol ineffective were discovered, upon further investigation, to have been flawed in some manner or other.

Recent research conducted by Dr. Belluscio has demonstrated consistent results with hCG. Records show that his clinic has used the sublingual hCG approach on 6,540 patients to date. This reliable and effective method for obesity management has been validated by appropriate double-blind studies. According to Dr. Belluscio: "Results are not surpassed by any other modality of obesity therapy."[18]

Most everyone can benefit from hCG. Whether you are struggling to lose resistant belly fat or are seriously overweight or obese, as long as you precisely follow Dr. Simeons' hCG program in conjunction with his specific low-caloric diet then success is guaranteed.

The tremendous proven success with the loss of 15-20 pounds of stored fat reserves on a 23-day protocol of hCG or up to 34 pounds if you extend the program to 40 days, has medical doctors, chiropractors, naturopaths and other natural health practitioners convinced that Dr. Simeons' hCG protocol is truly an effective solution to the obesity epidemic.

Cleansing the Body with the hCG Program

A little appreciated fact about the hCG program is the benefit derived from following the dietary protocol. In addition to helping the body release stored fat reserves, it also has the added benefit of a cleansing diet.

Few people actually make the connection between their symptoms or imbalances such as high blood pressure, high cholesterol, high blood sugar, pain, depressed moods, insomnia, arthritis, skin conditions and the modern, junk food diet. Let's face it. We were never designed to have radiant health while daily consuming coffee, alcohol, sugar, processed foods, ice cream, cookies, French fries, food additives…and the like! To add insult to injury, many of these foods actually cause cravings. Unknowingly people are caught in the vicious circle of eating toxic foods, which make them crave more of the same toxic foods. You become a prisoner of your cravings.

The genius of the hCG program is that you must follow a healthy, sugar-free, carb-free, alcohol-free, processed food-free, soda-free program in order to succeed on the protocol.

So you might say, you have just committed to a cleansing program as well.

In no time at all, most people are amazed and delighted to experience so many positive changes occurring. Aches and pains disappear. Allergies clear up. Headaches are gone. Pain, inflammation and arthritis are profoundly reduced or eliminated. Sleep and sleep apnea improves. Energy replaces fatigue. Skin begins to glow! All the key barometers of health such as blood pressure, blood sure, triglycerides and cholesterol move in the direction of optimal levels.

The light bulb then goes off! Feeling so terrible really is linked to poor food choices! A great big bonus of the hCG program is its ability to stop cravings. Real freedom is to be free of cravings. Then it is easy and effortless to make the best choices for your health and well-being for the long term.

The hCG program becomes your portal to optimal wellness.

The Controversy Over hCG

To date, hCG is not approved by the FDA for obesity treatment. After Dr. Simeons first published reports of his protocol for use of hCG in the treatment of obesity, his preliminary communication was followed by a myriad of reports, some of them favoring the use of hCG, and others criticizing the procedure.

Finally, and after a series of double-blind tests, the FDA concluded the method bears no utility for obesity therapy.

The FDA states: "hCG has no known effect on fat mobilization, reducing appetite or sense of hunger, or body fat distribution. hCG has not been demonstrated to be an effective adjunct therapy in the treatment of obesity and does not increase fat losses beyond that resulting from caloric restriction."

The FDA forced pharmaceutical companies to include in their hCG leaflets a paragraph stating that hCG was of no use in the management of obesity. The FDA parameters for approving drugs for obesity treatment specify that more weight should be lost with use of drug vs. placebo.

The research studies (including Simeons' research) found that the group receiving the hCG with the diet had little to no hunger (while the non-hCG group was starving). More importantly, the hCG groups lost dramatically more inches, and had a reshaping of their bodies. Furthermore, those who used hCG kept the weight off; whereas, low-calorie dieters tend to gain the weight back once they are off the diet. At the end of the day, the result from the hCG experience speaks for itself.

What counts most of all in regards to healthy and effective weight loss is what kind of weight is being lost. In the case of the hCG protocol, only the abnormal fat reserves are released; not subcutaneous fat, not normal fat, and not muscle mass. These distinctions were not addressed by the FDA. And, unfortunately, the FDA missed the important and most relevant feature of the Simeons' protocol.

While the FDA continues to maintain that hCG is of no use in the management of obesity, experience of patients throughout the years has proven that weight loss and the quality of weight loss (reduction of fat) validates that it does indeed work.

In fact, Dr. Simeons did decades of research with over ten thousand patients that showed hCG was very successful for permanent weight loss. Subsequent research has shown that hCG plus a low-calorie diet has numerous advantages over a low-calorie diet alone. His results were published in the journal *Lancet* in 1954. [17]

And then there is the issue of economics, hCG is not patentable. This poses a major drawback for pharmaceutical companies, which are only interested in a patentable drug. At present there are no patents for the various forms of hCG delivery i.e. injectable or sublingual. And it is also important to note that these forms of hCG must be prescribed and overseen by a medical doctor. The homeopathic version of hCG, however, is a safe, natural remedy created by using traditional homeopathic formulations and does not require FDA approval or medical supervision.

Dr. Daniel Belluscio, a world authority on hCG, explains the biases and prejudices regarding the medical profession's lack of understanding regarding hCG.

> I am concerned that well-trained and reputable health-care professionals may sustain that hCG can cause cancer, hirsutism, water retention and allergic reactions. But still more amazing is the fact that pharmaceutical firms must include in their hCG information leaflets that hCG has to be held accountable for all these side effects. If hCG is indeed responsible for all those side effects, pregnancy should be considered a high-risk condition, since hCG is produced in enormous amounts during pregnancy (up to 1,000,000 IU daily). The logical conclusion is that many pregnant women should become hirsute, develop cancer, or be seriously edematized.

> In reality hCG is a safe substance. When used properly, and in the amounts indicated, it has no side effects and provides no unfavorable results. The vast majority of reported complications are related to the simultaneous overuse of hCG and hCG (Human Menopausal Gonadotrophin) to provoke superovulation in infertility cases.

> It is clear that the success of hCG for weight loss relies totally on adhering strictly to the proper hCG protocol as well as the specific very low calorie diet meticulously created and proven by Dr. Simeons.

A Cautionary Note

While it has been demonstrated that most people experience exceptional results using the hCG protocol, there are some pre-existing conditions that are contraindicated for this program.

---

hCG Contraindications

1. Systemic Infections or diseases causing protein wasting.

2. Unstable angina, myocardial infarction (within three months), malignant dysrhythmias, prolonged QT syndromes or history of syncopy due to cardiac causes.

3. Recent or recurrent cerebrovascular accidents and/or transient ischemic attacks.

4. Documented significantly decreased renal function.

5. Severe or end-stage liver disease.

6. History of bulimia nervosa or anorexia nervosa.

7. Coumadin Therapy

8. Any Cancer, active or inactive.

9. Pregnancy and mothers who are nursing.

10. Uncontrolled Diabetes (A1C in excess of 7.0).

11. HIV

12. Hashimoto Graves Disease.

13. Gout

Possible Side-Effects of hCG

Although not common, some people have reported the following side effects:

1. Constipation

2. Hunger

3. Insomnia

4. Breast swelling

5. Leg and muscle cramps

6. Fatigue

7. Changes in the menstrual cycle

8. Hypoglycemia (low-blood sugar symptoms such as headaches, dizziness, hunger, irritability).

Leg and muscle cramps can be alleviated by taking 400 mg of potassium per day during the protocol. If that does not work after two days, take 8 tablets a day of a high potency multi-vitamin.

Always consult with your medical doctor before embarking upon this program and be sure that you are monitored throughout the protocol.

The Constipation Dilemma:
Keep on the Move

A commonly reported side effect is constipation. How do you know if you're constipated? Rule of thumb, you always need to have at least one bowel movement a day. Anything less than that falls into the constipation category.

Here are some tips to help keep you moving!

- Water…Water…Water. Keep hydrated. During all the phases you should drink at least half your body weight in ounces (200 pounds equals 100 ounces). 3 quarts of water or 12 eight-ounce glasses of water will facilitate in digestion process and flushing out of toxins and fat found in kidney. It is absolutely critical to drink the required amount of water daily while on this program for optimal success.

- Add more fiber. Mixing soluble fiber to a glass of water is also a good way to prevent constipation. Some effective fibers are psyllium seeds, PGX (Konjac root), acacia fiber. None of these have any calories.

- Constipation may also be treated with natural colon cleansing methods with gentle herbal laxatives. Be gentle. Do not use strong purgatives.

- Magnesium. A little secret for constipation is magnesium citrate, which can be purchased from your local pharmacy or health food store. Magnesium citrate absorbs increased water in your intestines, which causes peristalsis to occur. Since your intestines will be absorbing this excess water from your body it is very important to drink plenty of water after taking magnesium citrate. It's best taken at bedtime.

- Colonic Therapy. You might also consider going to a colonic therapist. Even if you were not constipated, a colonic therapist would support your hCG program because it is a great way to detoxify the body.

The hCG Choices: The Prescribed Hormone (Injectable or Sublingual) or Homeopathic

Dr. Simeons' original program was based upon daily injections of 125 IU of the hCG hormone. The growing interest in hCG has also provided other forms of delivery. There are now versions of the hCG hormone that are available as sublingual drops. Since hCG is a prescribed drug, any version of it must be administered by a medical doctor.

It is not recommended that a consumer purchase their own hCG hormone through the internet for several reasons. First of all, unless properly mixed and preserved, the mixture can become contaminated. That's the last thing you want to be injecting into your body. The other concern, is regarding the purity of the product. Since most forms of the injectable hormone is are obtained from overseas, mostly China, you cannot be guaranteed of its purity. Thirdly, most people have neither the experience nor the desire to do an intramuscular injection on themselves.

Since hCG has become so popular, another option has been created using a homeopathic remedy. A homeopathic remedy creates the same environment in the body as when the actual substance is given. It is taken as sublingual drops that are placed under the tongue.

The success and efficacy of the homeopathic hCG is demonstrated by the fact that it is now a commonly used homeopathic, probably one of the most widely used homeopathics ever created at this point. All observational data validates the effectiveness of the homeopathic version of hCG provided that the exact Simeons' protocol is followed. Homeopathic hCG does not require a prescription, which makes it a more affordable option.

A word of caution is also necessary regarding the choice of a homeopathic remedy. Be sure that it is made in an FDA approved laboratory and in a traditional manner. Secure the homeopathic remedy from a reliable and professional source.

Whichever form of hCG you should choose to use, it is important to ensure that it is of the highest and purest quality. It is also advised that you work with a qualified health practitioner to assist and assess you throughout the program. Many profound physiological changes occur, and it is necessary to be monitored by a health professional especially if you are presently taking medications for blood pressure, thyroid and diabetes.

A Word About Homeopathy

Homeopathy is the second most widely used system of medicine in the world. It has been the primary medical system of choice for a great number of people in other countries for many years. Homeopathy has been used for more than 200 years to help bring about healing and better health without the negative consequences and side effects so often experienced from allopathic medicine. Its popularity in the United States has grown dramatically over the last decade because homeopathy is effective, all natural and safe. There are no dangerous side effects with homeopathic remedies, and they can be taken along with other medications without concern for adverse reactions.

Homeopathic formulations function on the theory of "like heals like" and that a very small amount of the active ingredient brings about change. True homeopathic products have the active ingredients so diluted that they can no longer be detected by normal laboratory assessment. Since homeopathy is an energy medicine, the key ingredients actually exist as a unique energy signature or imprint in the carrier liquid that cannot be measured chemically. Essentially, homeopathic remedies work on an energetic level to produce profound physical and emotional improvements.

hCG Hormone Injections	hCG Homeopathic Drops
Effectiveness	
On average, a pound a day weight loss	Equally effective and can easily help shed, on average, a pound a day.
Benefits	
hCG injections produce consistent results.	The hCG homeopathic drops are diluted and hence, more powerful.
Fast absorption	Ready made and does not require any mixing job.
Administration	
Injected	Sublingual
Longevity	
The shots usually have an expiration date on them.	No expiration date.
Safety	
Infections, swelling and itchiness from injections.	No fear of infections, swelling and itchiness
Side Effects	
Shots may cause pain, lumps and muscle cramps.	No pain, lumps and muscle cramps.
Nausea, vomiting and dizziness are common with shots.	No Nausea, vomiting and dizziness.
Refrigeration	
The shots require refrigeration.	The hCG homeopathic drops do not require refrigeration.
Warnings	
Requires prescription.	Does not require prescription.
Needs caution while mixing the ingredients of injections.	Must not be exposed to microwave radiation
Presence of Physician	
YES	NO (Advised to work with health professional.)
Handling	
Mixing and administration of shots are complicated.	Easy to use.

A Word About hCG's Protection for Breast Cancer

The growing interest in the use of hCG for weight loss has generated a concern that it might contribute to an increased risk of breast cancer. Fortunately several major studies reported the exact opposite effect. In fact, clinical trials are presently underway testing hCG as an effective protection for breast cancer.

In 2005, Irma H. Russo, MD, the chief of molecular endocrinology at Fox Chase Cancer Center in Philadelphia, Pennsylvania presented the landmark study at the annual meeting of the American Association for Cancer Research. Dr. Russo's study was an attempt to recreate the protection offered by pregnancy through the use of hormones. The researchers gave pubescent rats cancer causing drugs to create breast tumors. Once this process was completed, the same rats were given one of two treatments for a full two weeks: 1. hCG supplements or 2. Estrogen and Progestin Hormones. The rats that had undergone cancer induction and treatment were then compared to control rats.

Her study showed that hCG activates tumor suppressor genes and stops cancer cell growth in animal studies.

The studies indicated that the animals that were given hCG experienced a reduction in the number of cells dividing. They also experienced an increase in the production of tumor-suppressor genes. The hCG also resulted in a decrease in the amount of cells that carried estrogen receptors. Estrogen receptors help most breast cancer cells grow. In conclusion, the hCG performed just like an effective anti-cancer drug. The hCG treatment resulted in similar genetic signature changes that were recorded as a result of pregnancy.

The hCG displayed definite anticancer effects on the subjects of the study.

Dr. Russo sees hCG as having a role in the future of breast cancer prevention. She hopes to see it used as a way to help women at high risk to alter their genetic signature to obtain protection for life from the ever increasing dangers of breast cancer. Her goal is that it will eventually be on the level with the currently in use Tamoxifen but with the added benefit of being a normal product of the body with no toxic effects.

At the 100th Annual Meeting of the American Association for Cancer Research in 2009, Johana Vanegas, M.D., a research associate at Fox Chase, presented findings suggesting that even a much shorter exposure to hCG can prevent breast cancer in rats.

Dr. Vanegas stated: "The ability to replicate the naturally protective effects of pregnancy against breast cancer will hold a significant public health value. In order to translate our finding into humans, a clinical trial with hCG as a preventive agent against breast cancer, is already ongoing in pre-menopausal women with no previous pregnancy."

There have been several follow up studies with prominent researchers from all around the world, which have all shown the same results. So, is there any truth that hCG is a risk factor for breast cancer? Not a chance. In fact, hCG is emerging as an effective and protective treatment for the protection and even potential, prevention of breast cancer. [19, 20, 21, 22, 23, 24, 25]

The Protocol, in a Nutshell

Dr. Simeons' hCG program is either a 23 Day Protocol (for those who have 15 pounds or less to lose) or the 40 Day Protocol (for those who want to lose 15-34 pounds), whichever you use depends on how much weight you would like to lose.

There are three phases that comprise the protocol. It is

imperative that all three phases are completed to receive the lasting benefits of this program.

PHASE 1:
Loading Phase

This phase consists of the first 2-3 days. This is when you begin to use hCG. Its purpose is to build up normal fat stores by eating a diet high in fats. Eat as much as you want and whatever you want.

The loading works with the hCG to restore any normal fat stores that may be depleted with excessive dieting. Also, it may take up to three days for the hCG to start working and so you cannot be on a low-calorie diet until it does. The emphasis here is on eating as much food as you can and consuming foods that are high in fat. If you don't do this, you may be hungry on the protocol.

During this phase, it is common for most patients to gain weight. This is a sign your body is rebuilding some necessary normal fat reserves.

The best foods to consume are healthy high fat calorie foods such as full fat dairy products, salmon, fatty cuts of meat, bacon, olives, nuts, oils, eggs, butter, olive oil, avocados, fish oil supplements, etc.

This is really not about overdoing a junk food diet. Dr. Simeons clearly stated that this was a time to eat a high fat diet, not a high sugar, high carb or processed food diet!

PHASE 2:
The Very Low Calorie Diet and daily hCG

This phase consists of the next 21 days or 38 days (depending on if you chose the 23 or 40 day Protocol). It is a 500 calorie program based upon specific foods in specific amounts, based upon Dr. Simeons' meticulous research.

Once on Phase 2, most people will average one pound of weight loss per day. More weight may be lost in the earlier part of this phase of the program, and possibly less in the later part of Phase 2, depending on how much weight you have to lose. Men usually lose weight more easily and more quickly than women.

It consists of two meals of 3.5 oz of lean protein, plus vegetables, fruits, and a breadstick or Melba toast. It is important to drink a sufficient amount of pure water daily.

No dietary fats are allowed during this phase.

Also all, moisturizers, lotions, and creams are eliminated. Your body will release less fat if there is an external source of fat being absorbed through your skin since whatever you put on the skin is absorbed into the body just as though you ate it.

Only gentle exercise is recommended.

Did You Say A 500 Calorie Diet?

This is the part of the program that raises people's eyebrows. While many people may be intrigued by the protocol and even consider embarking upon it, the thought of 500 calories a day suddenly stops people in their tracks. This is also usually the point that critics take exception in regards to the protocol.

Everyone knows that 500 calories a day is an unacceptable diet. This is true for every program EXCEPT the Simeons' protocol. Remember that under the influence of hCG in conjunction with a low calorie diet, the body will begin burning those stored fat reserves. And, one other point is important to remember, in the presence of hCG and a low caloric diet, the body will liberate 1,500-4,000 calories a day to be transformed into energy and nutrition.

Here is what Dr. Simeons had to say: "Just as the daily dose of hCG is the same in all cases, so the same diet proves to be satisfactory for a small elderly lady of leisure or a hard working muscular giant. Under the effect of hCG the obese body is always able to obtain all the calories it needs from the abnormal fat deposits, regardless of whether it uses up 1,500 or 4,000 per day. It must be made very clear to the patient that he is living to a far greater extent on the fat which he is losing than on what he eats."

This is the consistent experience of the thousands of people who have followed this program. Seeing is believing!

Transitioning from Phase 2 to Phase 3

At the completion of Phase 2, you stop taking hCG but continue following the restricted calorie diet for an additional three days. This is a time to eliminate all hCG from your body. If you resume a normal calorie diet without this washout period, you will gain significant amounts of weight.

PHASE 3: Maintenance Phase
(No Starch – No Sugar Phase)

No hCG is used during Phase 3

The maintenance phase is the time for the body to consolidate and establish a new metabolic set point for the weight changes that have occurred in Phase 2. It is an essential part of Dr. Simeons' protocol and must be followed to ensure permanent results from this program. This phase is just as important as your rapid weight loss period. In many ways this period is even more important when it comes to making your weight loss permanent.

During Phase 3 your body integrates the positive shifts and balances it has created during Phase 2. At this time your body stabilizes the weight you've lost, creates a new awareness and relationship to the foods you eat and sets the pattern for maintaining your new body size permanently.

Phase 3 is followed for the same number of days that you were on Phase 2, i.e. if you did 21 days of Phase 2, you would then do 21 days on Phase 3.

During this phase there is no calorie restriction. You can eat as much as you want of a whole foods diet focusing on a wide variety of vegetables, proteins, fruits, healthy oils, nuts and seeds, etc. Watch out for high sugar fruits such as bananas and watermelons. And go easy on the nuts!

There are two restrictions for Phase 3. You are not allowed to eat any form of starch (grains, potatoes, beans, corn, etc.) or sugar.

The No-No Foods for Phase 3

Pasta

Potatoes

Breads

Corn

Rice

Cakes, pies and cookies

Chips, pretzels, popcorn

Crackers

Candy

Sugared salad dressings

Ketchup and barbecue sauce

Cereals

Soft Drinks

Cashews

Peanuts

Bananas, watermelon, grapes, figs, mangoes

Honey

Molasses & Maple Sugar

Anything labeled "Sugar-free"

This is a phase where the goal to consolidate, not lose, the new weight you have achieved on Phase 2. You must not gain more than 2 pounds at this time. If find that you added 2 pounds, then Dr. Simeons recommended a high protein day called the steak day, which initiates fat burning, to get you back into the safe zone of 2 pounds, which is the weight you achieved at the end of Phase 2.

This is not a time to lose additional weight. Any weight loss that may occur on Phase 3 will be coming from structural fat, essential fat or muscle mass.

Also, Phase 3 consolidates the functional improvements that have taken place in the diencephalon area of the brain while you were on Phase 2. It establishes a natural appetite control and fat burning. It now becomes a normal part of your body's functioning. This replaces the abnormal functioning that, in the past, caused you to gain weight.

During the entire protocol, it is important to stay on all your prescription medications unless advised otherwise by your doctor. Although Dr. Simeons took his patients off most of their meds while on the protocol to make sure there was no interference with the protocol, he was able to closely supervise them at his residential treatment center.

If you are on blood pressure or blood sugar medications, it is imperative that you test your levels every day. Since the protocol will help you to regain normal readings, you must be sure to inform your medical practitioner that you are doing the protocol and have your blood sugar and blood pressure monitored on a regular basis.

The Importance of Getting Adequate Essential Fatty Acids and Protein

Once you have completed the very low calorie diet on Phase 2, it is important to replenish your body's ideal nutritional needs. Since no oils were consumed during Phase 2, this is one of the nutrients that must be resumed. This could be in the form of healthy oils used for cooking and or salad dressings such as olive oil, grape seed oil, flax seed oil, hemp seed oil, macadamia nut oil, walnut oil, coconut oil or sesame seed oil. You can also return to supplementing with fish oil or krill oil.

Since commercial salad dressings use unhealthy fats, sugar and chemical additives it is best to make your own.

The other key nutritional building block that needs to be included in higher amounts is protein. As a building block for all the key functions in the body from maintaining muscle mass, to optimal hormone production, to strong bones to enzyme product, to creating and repairing body tissues, to maintaining fluid balance, protein is a critical player for optimal health.

According to Dr. Simeons:

> Here too, the explanation is quite simple. During treatment the patient has been only just above the verge of protein deficiency and has had the advantage of protein being fed back into his system from the breakdown of fatty tissue.

> Once the treatment is over there is no more hCG in the body and this no longer takes place. Unless an adequate amount of protein is eaten as soon as the treatment is over, protein deficiency is bound to develop, and this inevitably causes the marked retention of water known as hunger-edema. The treatment is very simple. The patient is told to eat two eggs for breakfast and a huge steak for lunch and dinner followed by a large helping of cheese and to phone through the weight the next morning. When these instructions are followed a stunned voice is heard to report that two pounds have vanished overnight, that the ankles are normal but that sleep was disturbed, owing to an extraordinary need to pass large quantities of water. The patient having learned this lesson usually has no further trouble.

What's the Plan When You Complete the Protocol?

Here's the rule of thumb. Our body was never designed to eat a high carb, high sugar, processed diet. There is no diet on this planet that will allow you to maintain your ideal weight while you continue to eat such foods. If you go back to eating the same way that caused you to become overweight in the first place, you run the risk of gaining the weight back. In fact, it is pretty much guaranteed you will!

One of the benefits of helping to establish a healthy functioning hypothalamus is the freedom from cravings and a decrease in appetite. Also, the introduction of simple meals of fresh vegetables, fruits, proteins, healthy teas and at least 2 quarts of pure water reorients one's food choices.

Being liberated from food cravings, especially from carbs and sugar, is partly responsible for the long term success people achieve on the hCG protocol. Passing on the fattening carbs no longer requires an act of will power. The desire just isn't there any more!

Everything changes on this program. You are many pounds lighter, a couple of dress or pants sizes smaller, more energized, happier with yourself, and inspired to put a healthy program and lifestyle into place.

Meet Your Best Friend — Your Scale!

Most people dread their scales. It usually portends bad news in the weight loss department. In the past, the weighing in was a behavior most would shun. Who really wants to be reminded of the consequence of that Cinnabon splurge or the payback for being a couch potato?

The hCG program rewires those associations, creating a more positive experience. Who wouldn't feel great when you step on the scale and are amazed to find another pound or so has just disappeared over night!

During Phase 2 and Phase 3, weighing yourself every morning is a must. It will give you the feedback you need to succeed on this program.

When you complete the hCG program, let your scale (and be sure it is a digital one for greater accuracy) become your best friend, assisting you to maintain your ideal weight. Continue to weigh yourself daily for the rest of your life. If the scale shows that you went up a pound, then take measures that day to slim back down (increase protein, eat a day of low-carb food and lots of low-carb veggies, eliminate possible inflammation inducing foods). As long as you keep on top of your weight, you will not gain it back.

Starting a Second or Third Round of hCG

For many people going through one protocol may not get them to their ideal weight. This is especially true if you have more than 34 pounds to lose. If that is the case, then it may require several rounds to shed all those extra pounds. The beauty of this program is that, although it may take several rounds, the goal is assured. So, patience is the virtue that is required. It has taken some people a year and half to eliminate 120 pounds of extra fat from their bodies, but they have successfully achieved their mission. In actual fact, this program is the safest and fastest way for anyone who falls into the obese category to succeed.

In his book, Dr. Simeons recommended a 6-week break after the first round, followed by 8 weeks after the second round, followed by 10 weeks after the third, etc. This insures that your weight will stabilize before you make further significant changes.

If you don't wait the proper amount of time between rounds, you are at risk of building immunity to the hCG hormone. This would make it nearly impossible to lose weight.

> **It is important to note that the homeopathic hCG does not build up a person's immunity with multiple rounds.**

Chapter 7

Meeting with a Remarkable Man: Up Close and Personal with Dr. Simeons

The hCG protocol renaissance that is presently occurring is the legacy of Dr. A.T.W. Simeons. Many medical doctors and other health practitioners now recognize his pioneering work, as the breakthrough program that addresses the underlying cause of obesity. Although recognized as a genius, Dr. Simeons unexpectedly died in 1970 before he was able to begin his international tour to train doctors in his extensive protocol. While his work has remained, and is, in fact, gaining a tremendous amount of respect and success, there are very few people alive who have personally worked with Dr. Simeons. While his name is now legendary, there are few accounts of personal encounters with the man, himself.

Dr. Dan Koontz, who personally interned and was an associate of Dr. Simeons, is a retired Chiropractic Physician and Naturopathic Medical Doctor. He now consults with the nutritional industry and hosts the longest running live wellness radio talk show, *Healthy House Call*. Dr. Koontz has stabilized 50,000 diabetics using the hCG protocol, as well as helped thousands of others to lose weight!

The following is an interview with Dr. Dan Koontz who shares his experience with Dr. Simeons:

I first met Dr. Simeons in 1968 at a medical conference in Indianapolis. I was in the process of mixing up some cocktails with specific nutrients that basically blocked the harmful effects of alcohol. I was adding vitamin B complex, selenium, and milk thistle, chromium. While I was mixing this up, a gentleman came up and asked me what I was adding to the formula. I explained to him that I heard about this formula from an interview I had read with a famous doctor from Rome, Italy. I told him, "This was the famous doctor Simeons who had developed the largest weight loss practice in the world using hCG." We talked a little bit more and he said, "Well, you know you might want to consider adding choline, methionine and orthinine amino acids to that formula." I remembered that these additional nutrients were also mentioned in the article. He said, "These negatively charged molecules of the nutrients attract the positively charged toxins and neutralize themselves, thus, reducing the effects of alcohol."

To my surprise, he introduced himself as Dr. A.T.W. Simeons. He was also attending that very medical conference!

I proceeded to explain to him my interest in weight loss and that it was my plan to become a specialist in weight loss with the hCG program. I also told him that I had a particular interest in studying with him. It was that coincidental meeting that began this journey for me. It was really an exciting experience.

He suggested we had to go back to Rome, Italy and establish a research foundation. I told him my interest was really helping diabetics to stabilize diabetes through weight loss. He loved this concept. He said that he had done this thousands of times with his own patients. He also suggested that we establish a diabetic research foundation locally. In collaboration with Dr. Virgil Moss, MD, a very successful medical doctor, we did just that. Dr. Simeons worked with us from his hospital in Rome designing individualized, personalized weight loss programs with hCG as the heart of each plan. We would send him the information regarding the laboratory reports, examination findings of our patients and he would basically tailor all of our weight loss programs for each individual patient.

The hCG protocol was the core of the weight loss program that we utilized. The results were absolutely phenomenal. Over a period of two years, we stabilized over 400 patients. We could have treated a lot more but Dr. Simeons had requested that we keep it to a minimum since he was also in full time practice with his own patients.

The results were amazing. In every case we reduced their weight. Many of these patients were grossly obese. We put them through 40 day segments and in-between the 40 day segments of the hCG they did a 3 week stabilization dietary protocol of 1,500 calories per day with no carbs or sugar. Sometimes, if they were very overweight, they needed subsequent segments. They would average between a 30 and 40 pound loss during each 40-day segment. If we had to go back to a third segment, we would often allow 8 weeks or in some cases longer before we put them back on the hCG to make sure that the patient wasn't experiencing immunity to the hCG.

We had 100 percent success resolving their diabetes and metabolic syndrome symptoms. Only a handful of cases were not compliant. All the others were 100 percent successful. They not only got the weight off but also kept it off. One of the things that we learned from Dr. Simeons was his 'total' approach. Besides the use of hCG, he was a real expert in liver detoxification, balancing the thyroid, coordinating the thyroid function with liver detoxification and also colon cleansing. One of the things that often happens with the hCG dietary protocol is constipation. Whenever necessary, he would recommend senna seeds.

Dr. Simeons also taught me the key for successfully managing a patient who only needs to lose 5-10 pounds. After the patient loses their desired weight during Phase 2 (this usually occurs within 10 days), calories are increased to 800 to 1,000 per day until the 23rd day. This prevents further weight loss. The rest of the protocol is then followed.

Dr. Simeons taught that the hCG program could sculpt the body like liposuction because it specifically attacks brown fat. This is the most undesirable, abnormal fat in the body located around the waist, hips, buttocks and upper thighs.

Aside from being a brilliant doctor, he was so incredibly compassionate. He wanted to help as many people as possible. As a matter of fact, his ultimate game plan was to train me in his clinical approach and have me assist him with his practice in Rome, Italy. This would free up his time so he could begin his world tour, training doctors in his weight loss protocol with the hCG.

Working with Dr. Simeons was really a lifetime changing experience. His compassion was absolutely unbelievable. He was very realistic, very down to earth and just a phenomenal man.

Dr. Simeons was involved in ongoing research. He was such an inquisitive personality that he was always looking into other avenues to help his patients. He also felt it important to address the psychological aspects. It explained to his patients that they were experiencing a metamorphosis, a full lifestyle change.

Before any patient began his weight loss program, Dr. Simeons told them that they needed to reduce their intake of excessive simple carbohydrates, and sugar. He strongly felt they needed to understand this in order to achieve long-term weight management.

Dr. Simeons' program does not require exercise. However, he did suggest a walking program. Regarding exercise, Dr. Simeons recommended engaging in a regular exercise that each patient really enjoyed and to do it often.

Dr. Simeons found that all of his patients with long term weight challenges were experiencing various forms of degenerative osteoarthritis, orthopedic disorders such as chronic degenerative disc disease throughout the spine, degeneration in the hips, the knees, ankles, and feet. This was directly attributed to long term weight challenges and malnutrition.

To get the attention of the men, Dr. Simeons would warn them that obesity would reduce libido and put them at risk for erectile dysfunction. He said this really caught the attention of the men and helped them to be more compliant. It seems that warning them of increased cardiovascular risks, kidney failure etc., would go in one ear and out the other.

For women, he found that the subject of anti-aging got their attention and compliance. He explained that obesity contributes to premature aging and the breakdown of the collagen, thus more wrinkles.

With the hCG protocol, we can go a maximum of 40-day segments. We can also go as few as 23 days, as the minimum amount of time that it takes to make the shift in the hypothalamus, which regulates the distribution of fat. This was one of the keys I learned from Dr. Simeons. Once the first 23 days of the hCG is completed, the patient continues the 500-calorie per day program for 3 days and then we launch the 3-week program of 1,500 calories per day staying away from carbohydrates and sugar. When we continue subsequent 40-day segments, we have to have a longer break in between each segment before we launch the hCG again. This prevents developing a tolerance and immunity to the hCG hormone. Deviation from this program results in re-gaining the lost weight, failing to achieve successful goals and deflated emotions.

Despite my tremendous success when we began this program in 1975, it eventually fell out of favor with doctors. I'm not exactly sure why. Perhaps, because it was not approved by the FDA for weight loss. I am so thrilled that there is now a renewed interest in the hCG protocol all over the country!

Since 1975 with the collaboration of my associate Dr. Virgil Moss, we stabilized over 50,000 type II diabetics, in addition to thousands of others that were at risk. With hCG, I have seen so many people lose weight successfully, keep it off and eliminate their diabetic medication. They are then able to live longer lives, full of energy, enjoy fulfilling relationship and improved quality of life.

I just want to add that when I first began working with Dr. Simeons, we followed his precise protocol, which included injections of the hCG hormone. The hCG hormone is now prescribed as an injectable, as well as a sublingual form. I must say that I have also seen excellent results with the homeopathic version as well. All these forms work. With over 70 million American's being overweight, we need hCG in all forms to help stem this frightening health crisis and life threatening consequences of obesity.

I am thankful every day for the opportunity to have studied and worked with Dr. Simeons, one of the true geniuses of our time. I am so pleased to see that his work continues and more and more people are discovering the weight loss benefits of hCG!

Chapter 8

How a Medical Doctor Lost 115 Pounds

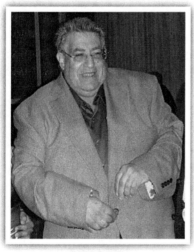
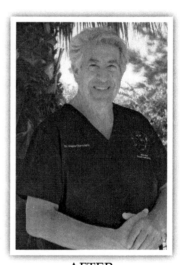

BEFORE   AFTER

Dr. Mayer Eisenstein is a man who is larger than life. A charismatic, brilliant, passionate integrative medical doctor, lawyer, radio host, lecturer and author. He is also an internationally recognized champion for many health causes. For many years, his large presence was also matched by his large girth. Dr. Eisenstein's, unending battle with weight finally ended when he discovered the hCG protocol. He shares his journey of physical transformation from 340 pounds down to 225 pounds, and is within sight of his final goal of 190 pounds.

Dr. Eisenstein was so inspired by the promise of hCG that he has incorporated a successful metabolic clinic into his Chicago-based integrative medical practice.

In this interview, Dr. Eisenstein highlights his personal journey as well as his medical insights on Dr. Simeons' hCG protocol.

Dr. Sellman: Dr. Eisenstein, you just accomplished something quite remarkable—you have lost over 115 pounds using the hCG protocol. It's all the more amazing because it's almost impossible to lose 100 pounds, especially in less than a year.

Dr. Eisenstein: Yes, it has been an amazing process for me. Less than 1 percent of people who are 100 pounds over-weight can ever lose any substantial amount of weight. I still want to loose another 30 pounds to get to the exact weight that I was when I got married.

In the past, I have tried everything in the world. Name any program and I've been on it. I'm convinced that the people who have tried many programs to lose weight are, in fact, the most dedicated, motivated people. It's not their lack of dedication and motivation that causes them to fail. It's because the programs are wrong; they don't work.

One of the things I learned from my research about the hCG program is that your body can't learn to maintain more than 15, 20, 25 pounds of weight loss at one time. Even if you're successful, which very few people are successful at losing 50 or more pounds, your body can't learn to maintain that new weight. It's been too drastic a shift. What happens is that the body craves to go back to the old weight. And it usually does.

On the hCG program, you can lose 15, 20, 25 pounds in one month and then, according to the protocol you have to maintain that weight for a set time (any where from 3-6 weeks) which is called the maintenance phase. In that phase your goal is not to gain, nor to lose. Then a month or six weeks later you can start the protocol again and you lose another 10, 15 or 20 pounds. This allows your body to learn to maintain the new weight.

This sounds so simple, at least the theory, but it's the most radical thinking I've ever heard. This is a unique discovery that Dr. Simeons made almost 75 years ago. His hCG protocol has made it possible for the thousands of people who are now following this program to be able to not only lose weight but also maintain their weight loss.

Dr. Sellman: I find this hCG program such an extraordinary gift, because I also lost almost 30 pounds and four dress sizes myself. I believe this program provides a new paradigm to help solve the obesity epidemic. While on this program, not only does your body radically changed but you also learn new behaviors, some habits, new knowledge and new life style choices that enable you to maintain the ideal weight as well as the improved health that you've gained. It actually jumps starts people into a whole new world of possibilities.

Dr. Eisenstein: That's exactly right. And learning is the key. There's nothing learned at a Weight Watchers, Jenny Craig, and NutriSystem, etc. I'm not criticizing these programs, but really nothing is learned from this experience. All you learn is to eat Weight Watchers food. Yes, you will lose some weight for a while. But the problem is, first of all, the foods that you're eating aren't the right foods. Secondarily, our body never learns how to adjust to the new weight. Even if you're successful at losing 40 or 50 pounds, you are never taught the critical things to do to maintain your weight and eating habits.

The most important rule for long-term weight loss is to cut out carbohydrates. The ones you should be eating are fruits, especially apples and grapefruits, and some salad. That's it! People ask, "how long am I supposed to do that?" My answer is very simple. How long? Just the rest of your life!

Dr. Sellman: Before I started the hCG program, I actually eliminated gluten grains from my diet. But I still was eating gluten-free crackers or gluten-free pasta, etc. And now after the program actually I lost my desire for all carbs. Just as you were saying, I'm not interested in them and I don't miss them at all! And as a result, I have been able to maintain my weight.

Dr. Eisenstein: My family has benefited tremendously from the hCG program. My wife lost over 70 pounds I've known my wife since she was 16 and she's thinner now than when I met her. My oldest daughter lost over 60 pounds. My oldest son not only lost 50 pounds, his waist went from 44 inches down to 34 inches.

Dr. Sellman: What's really amazing is that you've lost 115 pounds and your body looks firm and toned. Usually when people lose so much weight, their skin hangs on them and they look flabby, gaunt and old. But that has not been your experience with hCG at all, has it?

Dr. Eisenstein: The hCG absolutely tones the body and prevents skin folds and flabbiness. The hCG protocol, you might say, is a nightmare not only for the weight loss industry but also for plastic surgeons because if the whole country went on hCG, they would have a more youthful look and they would not have hanging skin.

Usually when people lose 100 pounds, their face sags, their skin under their necks hangs and their cheeks are sunken. This happens because on a calorie restricted program, collagen, the protein in your skin, which gives the youthful appearance, is being eaten away. Your body thinks it's dying, so it starts breaking down its protein. And that's where that old look comes from. But in the hCG program the fat is being released in your body. This toxic fat is broken down and used for energy. Thus, there is very little loss of muscle. And that's the reason why you end up having a youthful look as apposed to an old look in addition to al the other phenomenal benefits.

Dr. Sellman: Only the hCG program allows a person to release the stored fat, know as long-term stored fat or non-essential fat. On the hCG program, the body is never depleted of muscle mass nor structural fat.

Dr. Eisenstein: Exactly! And that's a really important point. We tend to think of fat as this amorphous blob but we now know that this long-term stored fat is a very biologically active metabolic organ. This kind of fat produces inflammatory chemicals and even hormones, like estrogen. So it is a major contributor to every kind of chronic illness that our society is now suffering with.

Dr. Sellman: In your clinic, you have every patient do a specific battery of tests to assess their progress on the hCG program as well as assess improvements in their health. What have you found?

Dr. Eisenstein: In my program I run several different tests: Hemoglobin A1C, vitamin D, the metabolic panel. But it turns out that the most important test that should be done is the vitamin D level. The reason is because it's easily correctable, by taking vitamin D supplementation. Low vitamin D levels have been associated with many health problems including metabolic syndrome and obesity.

The second test is called the hemoglobin A1C. It measures the percentage of sugar that is being carried by your red blood cells. The latest studies show that you want that number to be in the very low 5's or even in the high 4's.

You can only do it about every four months. Why? Because it gives you the amount of sugar being carried by your red blood cells and each red blood cell lives about three or four months. So after a four-month period you have essentially all new red blood cells. It gives you a measurement of what you've been eating for the last four months and how well your body metabolizes it.

I found that the majority of people have a hemoglobin A1C of over 5.5. Now what does this translate into health? Between 5.0 and 5.5 it's considered normal in our society, 5.5 to 6.0 are considered prediabetic. Having a pre-diabetic condition is a risk in itself. You have a double increase risk of heart attack, stroke and diabetes.

However, if your number is under 5, which is the goal I have for everyone, then your risk of diabetes is half of someone who's between 5.5 and 6.0. Now let's go up a little bit higher. Let's say you're 6.0 to 6.5. That means you are four times more at risk of what's considered normal, eight times the risk of under 5.

The bottom line is the majority of people are running 5.7 or 5.8, which means they are at serious risk of heart attack, stroke and diabetes.

And there's only two ways of addressing this problem. The first is by the use of pharmaceutical drugs, which won't ever correct the problem. The second way is the only way you can really do it. You must reduce the amount of sugar in your diet. Your pancreas will produce less insulin and, consequently, all your red blood cells will carry less sugar. Thus, your A1C will go down. You have now taken a major step in reducing your probability of heart attack, stroke and diabetes.

Dr. Sellman: This is really quite shocking. You're seeing high A1C numbers in your patients even when they have not been diagnosed with diabetes. So the hemoglobin A1C test is really a long term view of what's happening in the body. So, these patients are walking time bombs if they don't make some changes.

Dr. Eisenstein: That's exactly right.

Dr. Sellman: What is the Hemoglobin A1C reading with patients who have been on your hCG program?

Dr. Eisenstein: We found that four months later the average person is 0.3, 0.4, 0.5, lower that they were before. I'll give you the most dramatic case I had. The woman that came to me was about 40 pounds overweight. And she's been an insulin dependant diabetic for 15 years. Thirty days of hCG and her blood sugars were totally normal. She was no longer on insulin. She was an adult onset diabetic. Her doctor was astounded. He just couldn't believe it. He never had a patient who was insulin dependent for 15 years who no longer required any insulin. More and more of my hCG patients are getting this kind of healing.

Dr. Sellman: How can you be sure that people are losing only those toxic fat reserves with hCG?

Dr. Eisenstein: We use a technology that measures your water, your muscle and your fat. And we've been testing our hCG patients with it. We've observed that on the hCG program 60-70 percent of people's weight loss is fat! In comparison, if you look at all the other traditional calorie restricted programs, fat loss is between 10 and 15 percent. That's the reason why the hCG program makes you look so good. You are replacing fat with muscle and water.

I am totally convinced that the hCG program is the best way not only to lose "pounds and inches" but also to regain your most precious gift of all, your health.

Chapter 9

What Other Health Professionals Have to Say

Dr. Richard Delany, M.D., F.A.C.C.

Dr. Delany is a multiple board certified (Internal Medicine, Cardiology, Critical Care, and Geriatrics) integrative medical physician who has been in the private practice of medicine for over 20 years in Milton, Massachusetts. Dr. Delany has specialized training in both Anti-Aging and Functional Medicine. While maintaining a clinical practice that focuses on Cardiology, Internal Medicine and Preventive Medicine, he has also been actively involved in Complementary Alternative Medicine. He seeks out the best of both traditional and alternative medicine for his patients.

Dr. Delany is a dedicated and brilliant medical practitioner. He is also the consummate scientist. When a patient reported success with the hCG program, Dr. Delany's skeptical response was, "I don't believe that." So he set out to investigate it. To his surprise, he found out that it was true. If the entire protocol is strictly adhered to, following the proper diet, people get amazing results. They get to their ideal body weight without any abdominal fat. If they continue with what they learn on the program their extra weight will never come back again.

His very first patient on the hCG protocol using the injectable hCG was himself. It was a very positive experience. He lost 25 pounds!

His own success convinced him to offer this to his patients. The patients that do the best are committed to his program: they fill out forms weekly, they count calories, weigh themselves daily, drink the required amount of water everyday, monitor their energy, their hunger, they do very well. He also found that men tend to lose more weight than women.

Dr. Delany is convinced that this program corrects the hypothalamus:

> The way hCG works is by inducing the healing of the hypothalamus. When you do the specific diet and the hCG, whether it is in the form of cream, drops or shots, the body loses weight and contours change.

He has also observed the many ways that the hCG protocol has resolved health problems.

> It resolves metabolic syndrome. People who have dyslipidemia markedly improved. People who have truncal obesity markedly improved. Blood pressure medications are either eliminated or significantly reduced. Oral diabetic agents go away. Those with insulin dependent diabetes have been able to get off of the insulin. It doesn't cure people who have juvenile diabetes but it certainly cures the overweight obese diabetic. It gives people their energy back.

> It absolutely stops cravings. The reason the cravings disappear is because you cure the reason why the person is craving which is a dysfunctional hypothalamus. The patients who have central leptin and insulin resistance, all have metabolic syndrome. This corrects central leptin and insulin resistance. That's the cause of obesity.

So, it gets to the cause. No other diet available directs attention to the hypothalamus and its dysfunction in the abdominal fat.

Those are the two conditions that are not addressed by traditional medicine. The old model is 'energy-in, energy-out,' the ideal treatment for obesity today is reduction of energy in i.e. caloric restriction and increase of energy out i.e. exercise and behavior modification. It will routinely fail. Those three treatments do not correct the inflammation of the hypothalamus nor do they effectively get rid of the adipose tissue into the abdominal fat that causes the release of all the adipocytokines that causes insulin resistance, hypertension and diabetes.

That's why the late Dr. Simeons should be given a Nobel Prize because he found a way to address the cause of obesity. And my goal is to find out how it works and that's what I'm in the process of doing, slowly but surely. That's my goal: to find out why it works, on the molecular level and the functional levels. Then we may find other ways to help the hypothalamus. I think this is one way. I'm sure that there are probably other ways in the future.

Dr. Delany is adamant about highlighting the real goal of the Simeons' protocol.

The goal here is not only to get the weight down. It's to reset the hypothalamus so the weight doesn't come back. Now, I routinely see men and women changing. The women look better, they have a subcutaneous fat that's been restored to their face and they have remolded their body without any sags and they are just thrilled and they look younger. They routinely look younger. But if they don't reset the hypothalamus over the next three weeks, which is why the maintenance phase is a critical part of this program, they lose it.

Dr. Delany also had some interesting observations about the effect of hCG on the thyroid gland.

> I can tell you something about thyroid. As the hypothalamus becomes dysfunctional, it causes leptin resistance and insulin resistance at the hypothalamic level. It also shuts down; — this is my opinion — thyroid and sex hormones. As you heal it, they come back up again. So it's not uncommon that whatever dose of thyroid a patient may be reduced as they heal that access. Remember the access is the hypothalamus to the pituitary gland, to the thyroid gland, to the pituitary gland, to the testicles.

> I have read about 300 articles about hypothalamus. When you heal the hypothalamus, the body adapts. A dysfunctional hypothalamus will cause a leptin resistance and insulin resistance. It will create abdominal fat, which really give you lots of problems. It will also down-regulate your thyroid and down-regulate your sex hormone. Why do fat men, get low testosterone levels? One factor is in fact; they have a sick hypothalamus that is not giving the right signal. I would predict that men whose testosterone levels are low rise just as thyroid levels improved.

Dr. Delany lauds the genius of Dr. Simeons. More than 75 years ago, a man on a mission sought the solution for obesity and successfully found the answer. "The thing that fascinates me is this whole hypothalamus piece. Simeons was brilliant to come up with that. It is unique in this search for a solution and a root cause. It is just amazing that he pinpointed it and it seems to be valid."

Dr. Bruce Shelton MD(h) DiHom FBIH

Dr. Shelton has lectured extensively throughout the world and is the current President of the Arizona Homeopathic and Integrative Medical Association and the Dean of Bio-energetic medicine at the British Institute of Homeopathy. Prior to joining Deseret Biologicals, Dr. Shelton was the Chief Medical Adviser for Heel Homeopathics, the largest Homeopathic Company in the world. Dr. Shelton also currently maintains a private practice in Phoenix, Arizona.

Dr. Shelton knew it was time to address his personal weight issues, when he weighed in at 280 pounds. Arriving at 60 years of age, he realized that even the successful natural health program he was on could not save him from the consequences of carrying around so much extra weight.

He reviewed all the literature on it and six months later decided to finally try. And it changed his life...and probably adding many more years. In July 2009, he began his journey with hCG by using the injectable hormone form. With the help of his wife who kept him on the straight and narrow while doing this program, Dr. Shelton was finally able to lose 65 pounds after doing several hCG programs and eight months later.

As an internationally recognized homeopath, Dr. Shelton realized that the hormone form of hCG could be formulated into a homeopathic version. He was instrumental in developing the homeopathic hCG formula for Deseret Biologicals. Dr. Shelton presently uses the homeopathic hCG in his integrative medical practice in Arizona.

The following are his observations of the health benefits of homeopathic hCG for his patients.

> When you lose weight, your cholesterol goes down, your thyroid requirements go down, your sugar goes down, abnormal enzymes goes down, blood pressure

goes down. Arthritis seems to get better. Hair seems to get better. Fingernails get better, things of that nature. There are a lot of good pluses that go along with it. But basically, it isn't from the hCG itself it's from losing the weight. hCG just gives you the mechanism.

It's an amazing discovery that Dr. Simeons made about the diencephalon and how it releases the fat inside the fat cells that don't break down with normal exercise. I mean there is still a missing piece of the puzzle of what exactly is the signal from the diencephalon to the fat cells that make them do this, but nevertheless, it happens. It helps. It prevents diabetes, it prevents a lot of things that go along with high weight that you shouldn't have.

Dr. Shelton's experience also validates the effectiveness of all forms of hCG. He affirms that, "you actually reset your diencephalon so that your body stays at that weight."

Although most people will benefit from doing the hCG program, there are some conditions, which he believes contraindicated for this program.

Dr. Shelton elaborates when asked about the contraindications:

> Hyperthyroid issues—you cannot treat a hyperthyroid patient with this. You cannot treat a brittle diabetic with this. You should not treat a cancer patient in active treatment with this on chemotherapy. You should not treat someone who's just had a myocardial infarction not because it does anything to the heart except that it's a stress on the body to lose weight and if you put a recent heart patient through stress, you have to worry about it.

> We advise people who have hypertension on two or more medicines that they shouldn't be doing this because they're too brittle and we advise anyone else

with any other kind of health problems that are any kind of question that they need to be followed closely by their practitioner. They just shouldn't be given a bottle of drops and say, 'Go do this.'

We insist that patient come in and be examined once a week. We weigh them, measure them and see what's going on and draw blood if we have to.

He also addressed the concerns about the hCG-cancer link.

If the cancer is under control, usually it's not a problem. The one thing that a lot of people bring up the fact is that one of the tumor markers for cancer is hCG. If you have cancer, they do blood tests to see what your hCG levels are. I would say with the injectable form, you should do that, but with the homeopathic form, you don't build up hCG levels in your body. It's simply energy. And if your cancer is under control and you are well on the way to recovery and you're not having any problems, a weight loss program is a great idea and using homeopathic hCG is relatively safe. However, anyone with a difficult problem needs to be followed very closely.

Dr. Shelton is a living example of the power of the hCG homeopathic protocol.

Gloria Gilbère N.D., D.A.Hom., Ph.D., EcoErgonomist, Wholistic Rejuvenist™

Dr. Gilbère is a traditional naturopath, homeopath, doctor of natural health, eco-ergonomist, environmental health consultant, investigative health journalist, author of nine books and internationally renowned for her certificated wholistic skin and body rejuvenation (WSBR™) programs for spa and health care professionals. She is internationally respected as an authoritative influence in identifying the causes, effects, and drug-free solutions for leaky gut syndrome, fibromyalgia, chronic fatigue, and chemically-induced immune system disorders.

Dr. Gilbère was never overweight in her life until the convergence of a previous heavy metal poisoning with mercury exposure from her dental technician career days with the trauma of a near fatal accident. At that point her body went into a tailspin. One of the consequences of this time was a dramatic gain of weight. Suddenly, Dr. Gilbère found herself 34 or more pounds heavier and golf ball sized knots of stored toxins in her armpits.

> I believe what happened is all the toxins from the leaky gut that I developed circulated in the soft connective tissue specifically. And I not only gained 34 pounds immediately after I recovered from the leaky gut but I ended up with golf ball sized knots in my arms. Just above where the arm folds and there was nothing that we could do to get rid of them. We tried everything. And I couldn't get the weight off no matter what I did.

Totally discouraged about her intractable weight issue, Dr. Gilbère decided to try homeopathic hCG.

> The homeopathic hCG was like somebody handing me my life back. I didn't believe that it would do that. First of all I was concerned because I am borderline diabetic. Everybody in my family is diabetic and I've always managed it with diet. I was concerned that I wouldn't be able to do it because my blood sugar would drop and I wouldn't be able to keep that healthy level where you're not dizzy and light-headed etc. The complete opposite happened. Within 4 or 5 days of beginning my hCG program, I started sleeping better than I've slept. I had terrible problems sleeping since my accident and that was way back in '92. When I was on hCG I slept like a

baby. I am naturally a high energy person, but believe it or not I had more energy. I think more quality energy is a better word when I was on the hCG.

Over two protocols, Dr. Gilbère lost 36 pounds and three dress sizes! But something even more amazing happened to her. Her lumps under arms were radically transformed.

The left arm has no more lumps. They've all disseminated into the body. The body has gotten rid of them. The right arm, it used to be as hard as a golf ball would be. Now the lump is about half that size and it is starting to get little ripples on the side, which means that it's breaking up and the body is being able to get rid of it now.

Dr. Gilbère is now convinced that the homeopathic hCG can help improve many health conditions. She has incorporated this program into her practice, especially for her patients either at risk of diabetes or already diagnosed with it.

In all honesty the reason I put people on the protocol is because it's the only way I could get them to do it, is when they're so frightened about becoming diabetic. When their nurse practitioner or their medical doctor says, 'Okay its time to do something, you're either going to go on drugs or get serious about your diet,' and they're so frightened about becoming diabetic that I offer them this program. I say, 'Look this is what it did for me; my Hemoglobin A-1C was over 7 (which is the average of your blood sugar over the three month period). Mine dropped down to 5.4, which is unbelievable, because fewer than 6 are the healthy range. So that means that it completely got me out of that prediabetic state.'

When these patients went on the program, they also experienced the same benefits that I did. They lose the weight rapidly, they're not starving, and their blood sugar doesn't suffer. If they do the loading diet properly it

doesn't suffer. And their blood sugar A-1C went skyrock-
eting downwards not up. So that's been a huge benefit.
And then when they look and feel better and receive so
many compliments, they are encouraged to stay on it.

When asked she believes the hCG program is so unique and
so effective, she replied:

I believe there are a couple of reasons. Number one is the
fact that it does reset the hypothalamus. So everything
else we've tried—diet restrictions and all these fancy diets
—do not change lifestyle. And do not create metabolic
changes. They're not changing your body's mechanism
of how it deals with food and with weight.

And the second thing is that most of us have never in
our lives made our best friend the scale. I never weighed
myself on a regular basis. I always felt I could tell just
tell from my clothes. The truth you cannot.

Here's an example of what I mean. Recently, I was really,
really craving a big nice flour tortilla. Usually I don't eat
much gluten. On this occasion I ordered a big fish taco on
this wonderful organic flour tortilla with a little shredded lettuce and a little goat cheese. That was it. I gained
4 lbs the next day! By weighing yourself everyday, it
gives you a barometer of how your body is responding
to certain foods. It's been such an education for me and
my patients. I went back on having protein, as is recommended in the diet, and I lost those four pounds again.
Without weighing myself I would not have known that
I was gaining weight. I could have easily gone up 10
pounds or more before I realized what had happened.
So it's a really good way of being able to have a friend
on your side, a tool to make it a life style change not just
a diet.

Dr. Gilbère is now a passionate advocate for the hCG protocol.

I just think that it's the healthiest way I've ever found. As a naturopathic doctor, I can use Dr. Simeons' protocol with homeopathic hCG knowing that it is safe, easy, cost affective as well as helping to train you to have a healthier lifestyle.

Dr. Kendra Pearsall, N.P.

Dr. Kendra Pearsall is a Naturopathic Physician who has specialized in natural weight loss ever since she graduated from Southwest College of Naturopathic Medicine in Tempe, Arizona in 2001. She is the author of 9 books including: *The hCG Detox Diet and Dr. Mercola's Total Health Cookbook and Program,* She is also the medical editor of *The Hormone Handbook.* Dr. Pearsall's mission is to teach people how to achieve permanent weight loss with lifestyle changes. Her hCG website is www.enlita.com/hcgdiet

> I learned about the homeopathic hCG from another doctor who had tried both the injections and the homeopathic hCG and she found that the homeopathic had the same positive effects on appetite suppression and rapid weight loss that the injections did. Since then she has put all of her weight loss patients on the homeopathic drops and she said she has nearly a 100% success rate with those that followed the protocol.

> I started providing the homeopathic hCG to my clients and had everyone fill out detailed surveys after they completed the 6 week protocol. Over 88% stated that it was the easiest way to lose weight that they had ever tried and that they would highly recommend it to friends and family. Over 85% stated that their appetite was far less than usual with the hCG and 91% said that their food cravings and food addictions had significantly decreased using the hCG.

It is very rewarding to see the clients who have lost over 100 pounds with the hCG and who said that they had a new lease on life. I've had many clients state that nothing else worked for them but that the hCG diet did. One of the advantages of the hCG diet is that it is highly structured and people do tend to follow it to the letter. To be highly disciplined is difficult and many people are overweight because they lack discipline and structure, so this structure helps.

The hCG diet also requires that people weigh themselves daily during the diet and ideally for the rest of their life. Studies show that people who weigh themselves daily have a much higher chance of maintaining their weight than those who weigh weekly, monthly or not at all. Once people have lost significant weight on the hCG diet, they seem to be very motivated to continue taking action toward their weight loss goals and are pretty vigilant about avoiding behaviors that cause the numbers on the scale to increase.

Critics report that a very low calorie diet (VLCD) can be harmful because for one thing, it can cause vitamin and mineral deficiencies and muscle loss if stayed on long term. Dr. Simeons (the inventor of the diet) did not believe that hCG diet was a VLCD despite the fact that people were only eating 500 calories. His theory was that the hCG was able to signal lipolysis (the breakdown of fat) and that hCG dieters were actually getting thousands of calories in their bloodstream from this breakdown. He surmised this because he did not observe the negative side effects in his patients that are typically observed on a VLCD.

There are no research studies to date on the homeopathic hCG and there are mixed results of the hCG studies conducted with injections. Research needs to be done on the hCG diet comparing injections, sublingual and homeopathic hcg to placebo. To be on the safe side, I don't recommend that most people go beyond 24 days in a row on the 500 calorie diet unless they are being supervised by a health practitioner. Moreover, I recommend that people take a high potency multi-vitamin and mineral supplement and a potassium supplement (for potassium loss from increased urinary output).

Instead of fearing a temporary decrease in caloric intake on the hCG diet which mimics the normal periods of feast and famine our caveman ancestors experienced which kept them disease free and at an 8% body fat, we should be terrified of the modern lifestyle which provides 24/7 access to high carbohydrate, fattening, processed foods that are 180 degrees opposite to what our DNA is designed for. Periodic fasting and calorie restriction is the #1 recommendation by longevity scientists. When rats had their normal food intake decreased by half, they lived twice as long.

The hCG Diet also has a detoxification effect. The Standard American Diet typically contains wheat, eggs, corn, dairy, citrus, soy and sugar on a daily basis. These are highly allergenic foods that can cause food sensitivities. The hCG Diet is a narrow range of food choices consisting of low-fat animal protein, low-carb vegetables and an apple. People get off the foods that they are eating everyday which can lead to food allergies. Most people report having lots of energy and feeling very good on the diet. Also, many people have reported that their health symptoms disappeared on the hCG diet—a discovery also noted by Dr. Simeons. This is likely due to the detoxification effect the hCG Diet has and the avoidance of foods that may have been contributing to those symptoms.

Therapeutic fasting has been used with amazing success

to assist with overcoming disease conditions and increasing health and one of the reasons it works so well is because the body has more energy for healing and repair when it doesn't have to spend tremendous resources digesting food. The lower calories on the hCG Diet can provide similar therapeutic benefits for the same reasons. I think people would be wise to take the hCG Diet one step further and include a detoxification regimen on the diet that included a colon cleanse supplement, liver cleanse supplement, vegetable juicing, skin brushing, sauna therapy, hydrotherapy and enemas.

In conclusion, I think the hCG diet can be a powerful way to jump start a weight loss program because it gets people really motivated about the rapid results of losing one pound a day. After they finish both phases of the hCG diet, I think it's important to look at other factors of the lifestyle that may have contributed to the weight gain in the first place such as:

- Food sensitivities

- Brain chemistry

- Digestion

- Elimination

- Detoxification

- Candida

- Parasites

- High intensity interval exercise routines

- Emotional eating

- Hormone imbalances

I give my clients a questionnaire to pinpoint areas to address after the diet.

An ideal maintenance program is a slow-carb diet consisting of protein, vegetables, nuts/seeds and beans at most meals. Skip the grains, sugars and fruit. Eat this 6 days a week and on day 7 eat whatever you want, as much as you want. This hunter gatherer diet is what our caveman ancestors ate which scientists believe our human DNA is designed for.

This is the natural diet for optimal health and normal blood sugars. I also believe that daily exercise is very important. The latest research on exercise shows that high intensity interval training for only 20 minutes at a time can produce outstanding results in increasing muscle mass and HGH (growth hormone) levels.

Lastly, I wanted to say that I have enormous respect for Dr. Sherrill Sellman who is a consummate health practitioner, researcher and author who has made tremendous contributions to helping people learn about and improve their health.

Chapter 10

Up Close and Personal with Success Stories

Colleen's Story

I have struggled with my weight all my life. Sure, I've done other diets and was successful for a time but, inevitably, the weight (and then some) always came back.

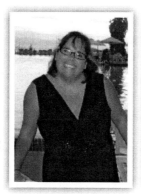
BEFORE

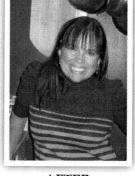
AFTER

I began my journey in October 2009 carrying a staggering 196.7 pounds on my 5'2" Rubenesque frame.

One day I ran into a friend and was stunned to see how fabulous she looked. It was more than her just being slim and trim, her skin glowed, her hair shone...it was an impressive transformation. I asked what her secret was and she told me about hCG. Like most, I was skeptical, but I couldn't deny her results. After considerable research and soul searching, I made my decision.

I did one round (Oct. to mid-Nov., 2009), following Dr. Simeons' protocol, and dropped 25.3 pounds and 36 inches (7 inches off my waist alone). Now, well over a year later, I'm down a total of 57 pounds and 55 inches (13 inches at the waist).

I had friends laying bets I'd never last. But the results I saw each day and continue to see, kept me committed.

And, truth be told, I have changed...my alcohol consumption is considerably less. Red and white wines are out. Quite frankly, neither taste that good to me anymore. Also, I've completely cut out the "whites" (potatoes, pasta, rice, bread, etc.) and with the exception of 1 or 2 dark chocolate M&Ms as an occasional treat, no sugars, either. Certainly no cakes, cookies, candy, etc.

The most important thing I've learned through my hCG journey is that a calorie is not just a calorie. I don't care what other diet pundits say. The scale does not lie. And 1,300 calories of lean proteins, leafy vegetables and light fruits is processed in this almost-50-year-old-body way easier than even a mere 500 calories from, say, a slice of veggie, whole-wheat pizza.

As the hCG program drums in, this is a lifestyle change, not just a diet.

Best of all, my doctor is especially pleased with the drop in my cholesterol, down 70 points from 268. My blood pressure is a mere 98/78 and my blood sugar is well below 80, down from 100. In fact, I am six month's shy of my 50th birthday and I do not take any medications

I'm maintaining fabulously. I owe it all to hCG.

Katy's Story

I'm really thrilled that I can tell other people about what I've done. This program has really changed my life. I'm 42 years old. I have a family with three children. And at the start of this program I weighed 183 pounds. I did the 23-day program. And I've had fantastic success. I found it very easy. I wasn't hungry and I've experienced some very large health improvements.

And so I had great success. I lost almost 18 pounds, which was amazing. And my body did change. I've got a fairly large bone frame so I didn't change a lot of dress sizes but my body did really change shape

I was originally diagnosed with fibromyalgia several years ago, which created a lot of pain in my shoulders. I've been sick for quite some years. What has been so unique for me is that I'm now pain free. All the pain has gone. For the first time in three years I can swing my arms above my head. I'm now even doing pushups with my personal trainer. It's something to be celebrated. This has had a huge impact on my family. In fact, my whole family is beside themselves. I have more energy partly because of the loss of weight, which produces a much stronger body but also because I'm not experiencing the pain. I do not have to sleep every afternoon, as I previously would have. I used to have to sleep between one and two hours everyday of my life in order to get through the day. I don't have to do that anymore.

And I've taken very careful note as I start to lose again of exactly what foods cause issues in my body. So I'm in that maintenance stage, I am careful to re-evaluate my health, which has been... actually another huge benefit of the program, you have these 21 days where your body gets a break and then if you're really careful about it you can learn a lot in the next 21 days, which I have.

Since I have been off the maintenance phase over the last two weeks, I had absolutely no trouble maintaining my weight. It's been stable which is great reassurance. Even though I was eating lots of food, my new weight held. This has been such a fabulous experience. I can fully recommend it to anybody. It's been an inspirational change in my life.

Ian's Story

Let me tell you a little bit about my experience. I lost 19 pounds on the hCG program. I must say I consider myself disciplined and I followed the protocol to the detail. I was quite surprised that during this low calorie period I didn't feel hungry. I read in the manual that consuming low calories while taking the homeopathic hCG, the long term stored fat would be burned and my body would get adequate calories to sustain my energy levels. I found this to be true, which was just remarkable.

Some people are afraid that this program will be too hard to follow, especially when they go out to a restaurant. Well, that happened several times to me and I'm thrilled that I just ordered off the menu. I just ordered chicken breast and a salad without any dressing and just had water with my meal and some herbal teas.

The protocol has completely changed my awareness as to food that I now consume. And I might add that I've maintained the weight that I've lost. I've not put on any more weight. I've changed my eating habits and that's the really significant thing. I don't have cravings any more. I used to be an ice cream addict but have now I lost all my cravings for it.

I did the protocol together with my wife. She has changed her cooking. We now eat a low carbohydrate diet. I feel more energetic. I think it's increased my self-esteem. I've even downloaded an App on my iPhone where I continue to weigh myself every day and make sure that I am eating the right foods and maintaining the weight that I fought hard to lose.

And of course the other benefit is that I can now buy some new trousers and be more fashionable!

Dan's Story

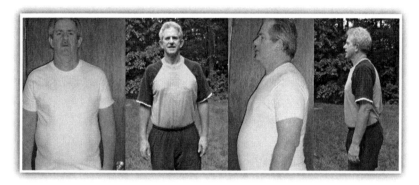

I was in a period in my life when I was in a weight gain. I was just gaining and gaining and gaining. All of a sudden up I woke and realized I had to do something. I didn't feel good. I was so uncomfortable and nothing fit me any more. I had no energy. I was just blasé, sitting around doing nothing activity wise. Looking back on it, it was a dark time.

After two protocols I was down to 215 pounds—so that's a total of 68 pounds. But probably the most noticeable thing to everybody on the planet was the inches. I lost a total of 54 inches!

After I lost all those pounds and inches, people didn't recognize me. I had an experience at Thanksgiving where a person that I had many conversations with in the past just stood there looking at me. He really didn't know who I was!

I also turned into the energizer bunny. I started training for a century ride. I was riding 100 miles a week.

This program also changed my attitude towards food. I'm very low carb and do my best to avoid all sugar. The experience really opened my eyes to the importance of what you put into your body and how to make smart choices.

Lori's Story

Weight loss has always been a life long struggle for me. For the past 15 years, I have been struggling with a major weight program. I have tried every diet out there with little or no success. The hCG program is first program that has ever been successful for me. Not only that—it has changed my whole perspective on eating, diet and exercise.

Before starting the program my weight had ballooned up to 320 pounds and I was a size 28. It is now a year and half after I began the hCG program and six rounds of the hCG protocol later. I am down 125 pounds and I am presently a size 16! I also lost 99 ½ inches! What's even more incredible is that my body has stayed toned.

I have had amazing health benefits, which I noticed within the first week of starting the program. My energy increased, my breathlessness was gone, my pain is gone, and the dark circles under my eyes are gone. My moods have totally changed. I am so much happier with life and myself. I just feel amazing!

My eating preferences have totally changed. I prefer vegetables, fruits and proteins. Before I would always crave carbs and sugars. But what is really amazing, since following this program I no longer have any desire for them. I make much healthier choices. I always keep healthy snacks with me so I don't have an excuse to grab something that isn't good for me.

What I want to say most of all is that this experience has been absolutely life altering. I look forward to maintaining this healthy lifestyle for the long term!

Kathy's Story

As a person whose inner compass is programmed to count my blessings, I'm thrilled to sing the praises of hCG; one of mother nature's little miracles! In my two year history with hCG, I was privileged to be engaged in the personal journey of seven people, all of whom lost considerable weight. Even more importantly, they learned for, perhaps, the very first time that they could actually choose health as opposed to bodies in chaos. I watched in joy as the scale became our new best friend. Collectively my husband and I lost 55 pounds; Stephen and Kristin C., 64 pounds; Sallie L. lost 25 pounds; Paula R. lost 20 pounds; Kathy C. lost 15 pounds; while Suzanne B. lost over 40 pounds. Pretty impressive results, I think!

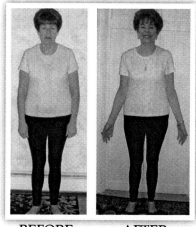

BEFORE   AFTER

Our miracles were all unique. Some managed to abandon blood sugar and blood pressure meds, while others were able to suspend antidepressants. One blessed soul became sober for the first time in years. But what was universal to us all was the opportunity to champion each and every day as we reaped the fruits of our labors. HCG broke the downward spiral of defeat and replaced it with a renewed spirit of optimism and anticipation of a new way of looking at and treating our bodies. What most excited me was the tenacious resolve of each participant to want to learn more and maintain the level of vibrancy and cleanliness that we all experienced. My "lending library" of natural medicine has never been the same!

Life is full of lessons for us all and certainly the hCG experience was a giant step in the direction of asking important questions about our bodies. The ability of hCG to open our minds and souls to new ways to wellness is a gift beyond measure. Thank you, hCG for finding us and bestowing on us so many unanticipated blessings!

Chapter 11
Frequently Asked Questions

What is the hCG Diet?

Dr. A.T.W. Simeons, a specialist on obesity and weight regulation, introduced a program that has helped many people overcome weight loss resistance. The program utilizes a natural hormone that is produced in the bodies of both men and women. It is also made during pregnancy. The program uses a natural hormone that is called, Human Chorionic Gonadotropin (hCG). Dr. Simeons' theory is that hCG causes the hypothalamus area of the brain to trigger a release of abnormal fat stores. When administered in relatively small doses and coupled with a very low calorie diet, people routinely report to us a loss up to 1 to 2 pounds per day. hCG has helped thousands of people lose those stubborn pounds. In addition to weight loss, many patients who have completed the hCG program also experienced many other health benefits, including a drop in cholesterol, blood pressure and blood sugar.

What is the Hypothalamus?

The hypothalamus is a part of the diencephalon area of our brain. This is the vital part of the brain which controls all of the autonomic functions of the body, including breathing, heart beat, digestion, sleep and the complex functions of the endocrine system. One of the many functions of the endocrine system is regulation and control of your metabolism and weight.

Does hCG work for everyone?

It works the same for men and women. The average that most people on this program report is a loss between 0.5 to 1 pound per day, claiming that it is the only program where they have been able to keep the weight off afterward. However, as with any drug or medication, or even with food (e.g., allergies), there is individual variation in its efficacy. Everyone is familiar with the fact that doctors often have to change people's medications because they don't respond as expected. Even though, hCG is effective for the great majority of people who will try it, there is logically no promise that it will work for everyone, every time.

How does hCG help me lose weight?

hCG appears to act on the hypothalamus, signaling the body to release stored fat into the bloodstream where it is then available to be used by the cells for nourishment. This alone will not cause weight loss though, unless you reduce your food intake. This forces the body to use the mobilized fat from the bloodstream. hCG causes the release of abnormal fat without affecting structural fat and muscle tissue. Which means you lose in those stubborn areas—hips, thighs, buttocks and upper arms!

Do I have to follow a special diet while I take hCG?

Yes. You must follow the entire hCG Diet Protocol as described in Dr. Simeons' manuscript, "Pounds and Inches: A New Approach to Obesity," where he outlines a special 500-calorie-per-day diet that was tested on thousands of patients. hCG is only effective for weight loss if it is taken while strictly following Dr. Simeons' hCG Diet Protocol, including the 500 calorie diet. Taking hCG alone (without the diet) will not cause you to lose weight. hCG takes effect when you reduce your food intake so that the mobilized fat will be used for your body's energy needs. If you fail to follow the diet you will fail to lose weight. If you only follow the diet without taking hCG, you are simply starving yourself because there is no fat in the bloodstream to burn. Simply put, both are required.

What food am I allowed to eat?

The hCG diet is balanced, unlike many extreme "fad" diets out there. It consists of a healthy variety of protein, vegetables and fruit, with a small amount of starch. You eat them in specific portions and combinations as outlined by Dr. Simeons. Allowed proteins are veal (low grade), beef (95% lean whole cuts), chicken breast (boneless, skinless), crab, crayfish, lobster, shrimp, and any fresh, white-fleshed fish. Allowed vegetables are asparagus, beet greens, cabbage, celery, chard, chicory greens, cucumber, fennel, green salad, onion, red radishes, spinach, and tomato. Allowed fruits are apples, strawberries, oranges, and grapefruit. Limited starches include grissini (breadstick) or Melba toast. Vegetarian protein substitutions (may slow weight loss) are a protein shake, egg (1 whole + 3 egg whites), cottage cheese or fat-free milk.

Is it healthy to lose about a pound a day?

Normally it is not healthy to lose about a pound a day on a very low calorie diet because it induces a starvation state in the body and will break down muscle and slow the metabolism. However, losing a pound a day on a low calorie diet while using hCG is a different story. hCG research studies have shown that those who used hCG plus the diet had lower body fat and higher muscle mass than those who did the low calorie diet alone. Also, hCG dieters have much lower rates of feeling hungry or starving versus those who do the diet by itself.

My doctor says that this won't work and is not safe.

Has your doctor tried the protocol? Thousands of medical doctors around the world over the last 60 years have treated hundreds of thousands of patients and have reported that the long term success rate appears to be higher than other weight loss plans. Thousands of patients have given testimonials about their successful fat reduction and weight loss.

What are the side effects?

Although not common, some people have reported the following side effects: constipation, hunger, insomnia, breast swelling, leg and muscle cramps, fatigue, changes in the menstrual cycle, hypoglycemia (low-blood sugar symptoms such as headaches, dizziness, hunger, irritability).

How is Homeopathic hCG different from the hCG hormone?

Homeopathic medicine is a holistic system of treatment that originated in the late eighteenth century. Homeopathic remedies take a substance like a drug or herb and dilute and success them hundreds of time so that the electromagnetic energy of the original substance is retained in the dilution, but toxic side effects of the remedy are not. It is this electrochemical "message" that stimulates the body to heal itself.

Essentially, homeopathic remedies work on an energetic level to produce profound physical and emotional improvements whereas; the hCG hormone works on the physical level of the body. People have found no difference in results or effects between those who used the hCG injections and those who took hCG sublingually.

How should I store my homeopathic hCG drops?

Homeopathic remedies don't need to be stored in the refrigerator but you will need to keep them away from electronic devices such as microwaves, mobile phones and computers. You should also keep them out of direct sunlight.

If on a very low calorie diet, won't I lose weight no matter what? If so, why is hCG needed?

Yes, you would have rapid weight loss with just a low calorie diet alone. If you attempt a very low calorie diet without hCG, you are starving your body and you will probably be tired and famished and not have the energy to maintain your activities of daily living. People report that they do not feel hunger nor fatigue.

Is hCG safe for men?

There are no negative effects on the male endocrine (hormone) system. It has the same positive effects for weight loss in both men and women. hCG is also prescribed by doctors to enhance natural testosterone production while preventing testicular atrophy during the course of testosterone hormone replacement therapy. hCG is also prescribed to cause the body to produce higher levels of natural testosterone after an individual has lost his natural testosterone production due to excessive use or abuse of steroid drugs.

Does hCG really have a resculpting effect?

Dr. Simeons' research has proven that it does. Normally low calorie diets deplete the structural and normal fat stores and muscle mass causing a person to look bony, sickly with sunken cheeks. On the other hand, people following the hCG Diet report a whole body rescuplting effect.

For example, a person may have an area of the body (belly, thighs, buttocks) where most of the fat has accumulated and areas of the body that could use more padding (such as heel pain due to loss of normal fat in the heel). The hCG Diet can help redistribute the normal fat from where it is in excess to where it is needed. It can help your body slim down, look more toned and rejuvenate the structural fat and helps it from becoming depleted. This makes areas like the face, neck and hands look and feel younger and rejuvenated.

If I only want to lose 5-15 lbs. can I still complete the program?

If you only need to lose a small amount of weight you can still complete the protocol. There are many benefits besides weight loss. It is an excellent cleanse for the body, helps you develop healthy eating behaviors and can help people overcome emotional eating.

Will this protocol restore structural fat that may have been lost during years of severe yo-yo dieting?

Quite possibly. Dr. Simeons saw that many of his patients who engaged in severe on and off dieting for years had sagging skin and an unbearable pain in their heels which they felt while standing or walking. When the heels of the feet were examined, the patients were found to have less than normal structural fat around the bones.

Within twenty days of the hCG protocol, the pain completely disappeared. In follow-ups over many years, no recurring pain ever was recorded. This, Simeons believed, was further proof that the hCG, plus specific diet protocol, not only removes abnormal fat deposits, but also actually permits the body to replace important structural fat in needed areas. This occurs in spite of the low caloric intake of food and those who took Homeopathic hCG.

Should I stop my medications while on Homeopathic hCG?

You should never stop your medications unless advised by your doctor. If you have specific concerns about certain medications when used in conjunction with homeopathic hCG, you should contact your doctor or a health practitioner specializing in the hCG program.

Should I stop taking vitamins while taking hCG?

While Dr. Simeons was strict on eliminating most supplements while on Phase 2, there are differing opinions on this subject. Since Dr. Simeons' time, our modern diet has resulted in many people being nutritionally deficient. Therefore, many practitioners are recommending that their patients include good nutritional supplementation while on the Phase 2. Please consult with your practitioner regarding the best program for you to follow.

According to Dr. Simeons, you will find that through the fat loss, your body will be recycling vitamins and minerals previously stored in your fat for re-use. In some cases, vitamins may interfere with weight loss especially if they contain hidden sugars. You can resume your vitamin intake during Phase 3 of the program. The one exception to this rule is digestive enzymes and probiotics, which will assist your digestion during the program and are recommended.

I'm not sure how many vegetables I should be eating during Phase 2

You can eat as many vegetables as you want during Phase 2 as long as it remains with the 500 caloric limits. Here is a suggestion on how to measure this: Weigh out the 100 grams of protein (approx 100 calories), and then add your vegetables, apple (55-110 calories), melba toast (20 calories) for the meal. Weigh out the vegetables and use a calorie counter to make sure you don't go over the 500 calorie limit. The size of the portions will vary with each type of vegetable, so use a calorie counter and a scale and you should do fine. An average serving size of spinach only contains 7 calories, for instance, while a 4-inch long strip of celery contains about 1 calorie. Here is a calorie counter that may be helpful for you http://caloriecount.about.com.

My weight loss appears to have slowed down or stopped. What do I do?

Don't panic! If your weight loss has slowed down or stopped, this usually means you have hit a plateau. This is more common in women than men and is a totally normal part of the program. You will most likely find that your weight will remain unchanged for a few days and then the weight loss will resume. It would be a good idea to read the relevant section in *Pounds and Inches*.

I've cheated and my weight loss appears to have stalled. What do I do?

Cheating always has a price on this program! Depending on how much you cheated, it may take several days for your weight loss to return. Stick with the hCG drops and 500 calories until your weight loss returns to normal levels. Note that doing strenuous exercise to offset the cheating is actually counter-productive on this program. It won't help you lose additional weight but will put stress on your body.

I'm in Phase 3 and I have gained more than 2 pounds from my finishing weight.

First and foremost you need to read the section about *Skipping a Meal* in *Pounds and Inches* which requires you to do a Steak Day or a high protein day on the day your recorded the weight gain. However, if this pattern keeps repeating and you are not deviating from the Phase 3 eating plan, then it is possible that you are having a reaction to some of the foods you are reintroducing into your diet. If you have dairy or nut intolerance this can cause inflammation and seeming weight gain where in fact it is actually water retention. You would need to go back and check some of the foods you have been eating and remove them to try and ascertain then eliminate the problem.

I'm experiencing food cravings.

If you have been on a high sugar, alcohol or gluten diet for some time, it is possible that you will experience food cravings during the program but these usually pass within a few days. Rest assured that once you finish the program, you will be amazed at how little you want these types of foods any more.

I'm still hungry!

Here are some things to consider. Are you drinking enough water daily, especially a glass before a meal? Perhaps you need to increase the use of a fiber supplement. Use some of the allowed foods to be separated into smaller meals to be eaten throughout the days. Munch on some celery or cucumber sticks. Increase the vegetable portions. Tale a supplement that helps with glucose control.

What should I do if I get constipated?

Drink as much fiber mixed in water as needed to have a bowel movement. Drink fiber drinks six times a day (such as psyllium in water). Herbal laxatives, magnesium and enemas can also help. Make sure you have at least 1 bowel movement daily.

When is the best time for women to start hCG?

For women, the best time to start is on the first day that your period finishes. This means that you will most likely avoid having to stop the drops during the program.

The instructions in all the phases call for a large consumption of water and teas. Is this necessary?

The tea drinking is optional. During all the phases you should drink at least half your body weight in ounces (200 pounds equals 100 ounces). Drinking plenty of water is important in the treatment of the obesity condition and for the protocol to work effectively.

Do I need to eat organic food?

No, but you are encouraged to eat as much organic, pesticide free, locally grown food as possible because it is far healthier.

Should I run and exercise while completing the protocol?

Many people are able to continue their regular exercise program or some degree of their regular program. If you haven't been exercising regularly, the beginning of the protocol is not the time to start as it may be too taxing on your body to be on a low calorie diet in addition to starting an exercise program.

Dr. Simeons recommends only gently exercise on the program. You can do daily walking and other light exercise during the 500 calorie phase (10-45 minutes a day depending on your level of fitness). It is not recommended to do strenuous exercise during that phase as it may be too taxing on the body. However, if you are used to strenuous exercise, you can try it and see how you feel. Some people are able to continue their strength training and exercise classes on the protocol.

What can I do to stop the leg cramps I have been experiencing?

Take 400 mg of potassium per day during the protocol. If that does not work after two days, take 8 tablets a day of a high potency multi-vitamin.

What about pregnancy and taking hCG?

If you are pregnant or become pregnant during the hCG diet, stop taking hCG and consult your physician.

I want to do another course of the program. How long do I have to wait to start?

According to Dr. Simeons, it is important to weight six weeks before beginning another protocol if you have used the hormones. In some cases, people using the homeopathic remedy of hCG, can begin another round sooner.

Can I drink alcohol on this program?

Alcohol is strictly forbidden during Phase 2 of the program. Dr. Simeons suggests that a small glass of wine during Phase 3 is acceptable but you need to remember that wine contains sugar so you will need to closely monitor your weight changes the following day and do a steak day if necessary.

I'm at day 23 of Phase 2 and am doing so well that I want to do the 40 day program. Can I do this?

Of course. If you wish to continue your program to 40 days you should maintain the VLCD and drops for another 17 days.

Can I do more than 23 days on Phase 2 but less than 40 days?

Yes you can. You just need to ensure that you spend the equivalent amount of time on Phase 3 – Maintenance Phase. For instance, if you do Phase 2 for 30 days, you will need to do Phase 3 Maintenance for 30 days.

My skin is really dry. What do you recommend?

If you find that your skin is dry, you may want to try applying organic coconut oil to your skin, which should improve hydration during the program.

Chapter 12
The hCG Diet Recipes

The guidelines for the hCG protocol as created by Dr. Simeons requires a commitment to follow the program precisely for the time you are on it.

Although the kinds of foods may appear limited, there are so many possible creative variations on a theme.

With the help of spices, sauces, seasonings and herbs, you will be surprised how interesting each meal can be.

The following recipes offer some possibilities that will allow you not only to enjoy the program but also inspire you to make healthy choices from now on!

This is an exciting and transformative experience. Enjoy it!

Dr. Sellman and Frankie's Pantry List

Bragg Organic Apple Cider Vinegar
Bragg Liquid Aminos
Fresh and frozen spices
Sea Salt (good quality)
Ground pepper
Lemons, lemon juice (organic, not from concentrate)
Limes, lime juice (not from concentrate)
Garden Tube Spices (variety)
Cinnamon (organic tastes better)

Pure vanilla
Assorted vinegars
Hot sauces
Mustards, mustard powder
Bragg Organic 24 Herb Seasoning
Oregano
Cilantro
Basil, frozen and dried
Celery seeds
Chili powder
Thyme
Cayenne pepper
Tabasco
Coriander
Cumin

No soy sauce, (most soy sauces have gluten)

Gourmet Garden www.gourmetgarden.com makes a variety of fresh organic herbs as a paste and packaged in a tube for easy use.

Coconut flour can be purchased at your local health food store or www.swansonhealth.com

CocoPure Tea is available at (800) 290-0221.

Konjac flour noodles (Shirataki noodles) are available at www.miraclenoodle.com or www.konjacfoods.com

Stevia and xylitol are available in all health food stores or at www.amazon.com

These are just a few suggestions of things you may want to have in your pantry to make the protocol.

Frankie's Tip:

Preparedness is the key for success on the hCG protocol. Make sure your pantry is filled with all the right condiments and spices before you start Phase 2. Also double make sure that there is no MSG or sugar in the ingredients.

Explore the world of seasoning:

Taken from Suzanne Sommer's newsletter:

Basil is rich in antioxidants like vitamin A and C.

Black pepper increases the hydrochloric-acid production in your stomach, aiding digestion.

Cayenne pepper is a cardiovascular booster.

Crushed red-pepper flakes contain capsaicin, a potent anti-inflammatory.

Cumin primes the salivary glands and improves digestion.

Curry powder combines all the benefits of cumin and turmeric in one quick pinch.

Dill is a potent antioxidant and a good source of calcium.

Fennel boosts levels of vitamin C and contains anethole, a phytonutrient that can prevent cancer.

Garlic can help regulate the number of fat cells in your body and protect your cardiovascular system from disease.

Lemon and lime brighten up the flavor of plain water and boost your intake of vitamin C.

Mint can help you fight cancer.

Nutmeg can help you get sleepy at night.

Onion offers similar cardiovascular benefits as garlic.

Oregano is, pound for pound, one of the most antioxidant-rich foods around.

Paprika is an excellent anti-inflammatory and antioxidant.

Rosemary may be a weapon in the fight against cancer by preventing carcinogens from binding to cells.

Sage contains the same cancer fighting compounds as rosemary.

Tarragon can aid digestion and help improve heart health.

Thyme is a relative of mint and a potent antioxidant.

Turmeric has been shown in several studies to have anti-inflammatory properties and could help protect against degenerative diseases like Alzheimer's and heart disease.

Vanilla is not only a sweet flavoring but a stellar antioxidant.

Phase 2 Recipes

Refreshing Drinks

Flavored Waters
Flat or mineral water
Any flavor of Stevia drops

Creamy Cafe Coffee
Pure coffee (organic, if possible)
1 tbsp of milk (only allowed 1 tbsp each day)
Vanilla Creme and Dark Chocolate Stevia drops

Sweet Caramel Coffee
English Toffee Stevia drops

Lemonade
Water
Juice of lemon to taste
(only allowed the juice of 1 lemon throughout the day)
Regular Stevia (powder or drops) or Xylitol to taste

Grapefruit Virgin Martini
Juice of ½ grapefruit
Vanilla Stevia to taste
Sparkling mineral water & ice

Dressings, Seasonings & Sauces

Catsup
3 oz tomato paste
3 tbsp apple cider vinegar
1 tbsp lemon juice
¼ tsp celery salt
½ tsp paprika

¼ tsp mustard powder
Pinch of nutmeg and clove
Pinch of black pepper
¼ tsp onion powder
¼ tsp garlic powder
Stevia to taste

Dissolve spices in vinegar and lemon juice. Add tomato paste and mix thoroughly. Add additional lemon juice, vinegar or a little water until desired consistency is reached. Makes 2 or more servings.

Dijon Dressing
Squeeze of lemon
1 tbsp vinegar
½ tsp garlic powder (or fresh)

¾ tsp dried mustard
Pepper
Xylitol or Stevia

Add all ingredients to a covered jar or container and shake to mix well. Label with the date if you are storing in the refrigerator.

Ginger Dressing
½ cup white vinegar
2 tsp Xylitol
1 cup Bragg Amino Acids

1 tbsp minced garlic
1 cup water
2 tbsp minced ginger

Mix all ingredients and let set for about an hour. Also, you can marinate meat with this dressing and then grill.

Greek Seasoning Mix
2 tsp oregano
1½ tsp onion powder
1½ tsp garlic powder
1 tsp salt & 1 tsp black pepper

1 tsp parsley
1 tsp basil
½ tsp cinnamon
½ tsp nutmeg
½ tsp thyme

Grind spices in food processor or coffee grinder.
Store in air-tight container.

Dressings, Seasonings & Sauces

Mexican Cocktail Sauce
Picante sauce or fresh salsa
2 Serrano chilies, finely chopped

1 garlic clove, minced
Juice from 2 limes

Gently combine all the salsa ingredients in a non-reactive bowl and let sit for the flavors to combine at least 30 minutes.

Mojo Sauce
4 Garlic cloves, minced
1 Jalapeno, minced
1 large handful fresh coriander
  leaves, finely chopped

Sea salt and freshly ground
  black pepper
2 limes, juiced
1 orange, juiced
2 tbsp white vinegar
½ cup broth

In a mortar and pestle or bowl, mash together the garlic, jalapeno, coriander, salt, and pepper to make a paste. Put the paste in a glass jar or plastic container. Add the lime juice, orange juice, vinegar, and oil. Shake it up really well to combine. Use as a marinade for chicken or beef or as a table condiment. Yield: approximately 1¼ cups.

Mustard Salad Dressing
¼ cup vinegar (or to taste)
½ tsp ground mustard

2 tbsp water
Sea salt and pepper
Xylitol (as needed)

Place everything in a covered jar or covered container and shake well. Can be stored in the refrigerator.

Orange Ginger Dressing
½-1 cup champagne vinegar
2 tbsp minced or grated ginger

1 tbsp garlic
Juice of 1 orange or lemon

Put it all in a jar and let sit for about 8 hours before use so flavors can meld.

Dressings, Seasonings & Sauces

Pico De Gallo
4 vine-ripe tomatoes, chopped
½ medium red onion,
  chopped
2 green onions, white and green
  parts, sliced
1 Serrano chili, minced
1 handful fresh coriander
  leaves, chopped
3 garlic cloves, minced
2 limes, juiced
1 tsp sea salt

In a mixing bowl, combine all ingredients together. Toss thoroughly. Let it sit for 15 minutes to an hour to allow the flavors to marry.

Raspberry Vinaigrette
2 tbsp raspberry vinegar
⅛ tsp sea salt
Freshly ground pepper to taste

Whisk vinegar, salt and pepper in a small bowl. Drizzle over salad greens or chicken.

Spicy BBQ Sauce & Marinade
2 8 oz jars Mexican salsa
⅔ cup lemon juice
2 tbsp Worcestershire sauce
4 tbsp Xylitol
2 tsp salt
4 tsp chili powder
½ tsp Tabasco Sauce – (hot
  pepper sauce - ½ - 1 dashes)
1 or 2 dashes garlic powder

Whisk all the ingredients together.

Sweet 'n' Vinaigrette Dressing
3 tbsp of raw apple cider vinegar
Salt, pepper to taste
½ packet of natural sweetener
(Stevia or Xylitol) to taste

Mix ingredients in a small bowl then drizzle over salad.

Vinaigrette
⅓ cup apple cider vinegar
2 tbsp water
2 tbsp dried thyme
¼ tsp salt & ¼ tsp pepper
1 tbsp dried basil
¼ tsp garlic powder

Mix all in blender.

Dressings, Seasonings & Sauces

BBQ Rub

I shook about 1 tbsp or so of this on my eye of round steak for lunch, rubbed it down, stuck in refrigerator for 20 minutes and then tossed it on the grill. Yum yum yum. This also tastes great on chicken.

2 tbsp paprika	1 tbsp black pepper
1 tbsp Xylitol	1 tbsp chili powder
1 tbsp ground cumin	

Mix and store in air-tight container/ziplock bag. This amount makes enough for several uses. This is slightly spicy so be sure you're drinking your water.

Cajun Seasoning

1 tbsp chili powder	1 tsp onion powder
1 tbsp Hungarian paprika	½ tsp dried oregano
1 tsp garlic powder	½ tsp dried thyme
	½ tsp cayenne pepper
	½ tsp freshly ground pepper

Combine and store in airtight container.

Caribbean Chicken Rub

I simply mix this up in a ziplock bag, add 3½ oz of chicken, and then shake, shake, shake! Let it sit for 20 minutes in refrigerator before grilling/baking/broiling.

1 tbsp parsley	½ tsp black pepper
1 tsp cumin	½ tsp allspice
1 tsp chili powder	¼ tsp cinnamon

This amount makes enough for 2 servings of chicken (possibly even more depending on how much seasoning you like) so you can shake both of them up in the ziplock, cook both, and then refrigerate the extra chicken.

Dressings, Seasonings & Sauces

Curry Seasoning

1 tbsp turmeric

1 tbsp coriander

2 tsp paprika

1 tsp pepper

1 tsp cumin

1 tsp ginger

½ tsp cloves

½ tsp celery seed

½ tsp cayenne

Mix and store in air-tight container.

Mustard Ginger Hot Sauce

1 tbsp fresh ginger, grated
(ground ginger or Gourmet
Garden ginger tube)

2 tbsp yellow mustard

¼ cup vinegar

⅛ tsp chili pepper

Mix together.

Frankie's Tip:

This sauce is a great topping for vegetables, meats, chicken or fish. To use as a marinade, double the ingredients.

Sweet and Sour Tomato Sauce

1 can of organic tomatoes

¼ cup apple cider vinegar

2 tbsp fresh lemon juice

Pinch of garlic powder to taste

Xylitol or Stevia to taste

Sea salt (optional)

In a medium saucepan, mix all of the ingredients. Simmer for 20-30 min.

Frankie's Tip:

This sauce is very versatile. Use it to top cabbage, spinach or beet greens. Also for sweet and sour meatballs or stuffed cabbage. If you put shredded cabbage in it, it makes a nice soup. I sometimes add a dash of hot chili pepper sauce for an additional kick.

Emeril's "Southwest Spice"

2 tbsp chili powder

1 tbsp dried oregano

2 tbsp paprika

1 tbsp ground coriander

1 tbsp garlic powder

1 tbsp sea salt & black pepper

2 tsp ground cumin

1 tsp cayenne pepper

1 tsp ground red pepper

Combine all ingredients thoroughly and store in an airtight container.

Dressings, Seasonings & Sauces

Mock Shake 'n' Bake
½ cup minced dehydrated
   onions
¼ tsp coriander
¼ tsp thyme

¼ tsp red pepper flakes
⅛ tsp oregano
⅛ tsp paprika
⅛ tsp black pepper
⅛ tsp salt

Place all ingredients in food processor or coffee grinder. Grind to a powder. Store in airtight container.

Frankie's Tip:

Use this as coating on your meat before you cook it. Dampen meat, then coat. This is great on chicken, fish, prawns, and even steak burgers.

Mexican Salsa

Boil red tomatoes and one chili pepper. When tomatoes are soft, pull the skin off. Put the tomatoes and chili pepper in blender with plenty of water and lots of salt. Vary the flavor using any of the following: garlic, sugar, coriander, onion, thyme, and oregano.

Soups

**Dr. Sherrill's Quick
Chicken Soup**
Organic chicken broth or make
your own (check ingredients on
any brand you buy to avoid oils
and fats)
3½ oz chicken breast
Fresh garlic

Fresh coriander
Fresh parsley
Grated fresh ginger
Chopped yellow onion or green
   onions
Your choice of greens i.e.
   silverbeet, spinach,
   watercress, etc.

Pour chicken broth into saucepan. Add chicken sliced into small pieces. Add chopped cilantro, parsley, garlic, ginger, onion. Cook for 15 min. Add salt, pepper etc. to taste

Frankie's Tomato Soup

Large can of organic tomatoes

Can of the roasted tomatoes
   with sliced chili peppers
   (if available)

Can of tomato paste

Add Xylitol to taste

Fresh lemon juice

Can add protein (shrimp,
   white fish chicken or beef)

Herbs and spices to taste
   (coriander, basil, oregano,
   cumin – whatever you prefer)

Cook all together with as many flavors and spices as you like. Use Bragg's 23 spices, coriander, Indian spices (this is where you can add your own spin). Add Xylitol to taste as tomato soups often require a little sweetening. Use a little lemon juice so it becomes sweet and sour. Cook it for as little as 5 minutes to up to an hour on medium-low heat. For a variation, throw in a bag of shredded cabbage.

Cabbage Soup

3½ oz of chicken or
   lean ground beef

1 cup organic cabbage chopped
   into chunks

2 onions

1 celery stalk cut into ½ inch
   pieces

2 cloves fresh garlic

4 plum tomatoes chunks or
   2 cup chopped tomatoes

Water

Spices to taste: sea salt,
   celery salt, garlic powder,
   garlic salt, pepper

If using beef, brown in pot and drain off excess fat. Add all vegetables and tomatoes; add enough water to cover it all. Simmer until cabbage is soft. Season with spices to taste.

Cream of Chicken Soup

3½ oz cooked chicken

1 stalk of celery

2 cups of chicken broth

3 cloves of garlic

1 tbsp dehydrated minced
   onion

½ tsp dried parsley

½ tsp dried basil

Ground white pepper (to taste)

Sea salt (to taste, optional)

Preheat a medium saucepan over medium-high heat. In a food processor, combine first 7 ingredients and pulse until smooth. Pour into saucepan and bring to a boil. Reduce heat, cover and simmer for 20-30 minutes until flavors are well blended. Season with salt and pepper. Serve.

Frankie's Tip: Boil the chicken and use the broth for the soup.

Phase 2 Vegetables

Ginger Cabbage
1 head of cabbage, shredded
  or the equivalent pre shredded
  packages

1 tsp Gourmet Garden Ginger
  or powdered ginger
Xylitol or Stevia to taste
Sea salt (optional)

Set oven at 350°F. Spread shredded cabbage in a baking dish. Sprinkle the Gourmet Garden Ginger or powdered ginger and either the Xylitol or Stevia on the cabbage. Sprinkle the optional sea salt. Cover and bake 15-30 minutes depending on how soft you like your cabbage. You will love how this makes your house smell.

Frankie's Tip:

Make sure you have fresh or frozen spices and herbs in your cupboards and freezer. One of my favorite choices that I use in all phases is by an Australian Company called Gourmet Garden. It is sold in the refrigerator section near the produce in supermarkets. They come in assorted flavors such as ginger, cilantro, lemon grass and many other varieties. Each one is better than the next. Do try them. When using Xylitol or Stevia it all depends on the brand and your individual taste buds. Stevia can be very strong, so be very careful. Too much Xylitol can affect your digestion and make you gassy. Both are natural and plant based. Experiment with dosage.

Lemon Garlic Cabbage
1 head of cabbage, shredded
  or the equivalent pre shredded
  packages

1 tbsp lemon juice
¼ tsp garlic powder to taste
Sea salt to taste (optional)

Set oven at 350°F. Spread shredded cabbage in a baking dish. Sprinkle the lemon and garlic on the cabbage. Cover and bake 15-30 minutes depending on how soft you like your cabbage.

Phase 2 Vegetables

Sweet and Sour Cabbage
1 head of cabbage, shredded
  or the equivalent pre shredded
  packages

¼ cup Bragg Apple Cider
  Vinegar
1 tbsp yellow mustard
  (powdered is also fine)
Xylitol or Stevia to taste

Set oven at 350°F. In a small mixing bowl, mix the mustard, Xylitol or Stevia and apple cider vinegar. Spread shredded cabbage in a baking dish. Pour the mixture over the cabbage. Cover and bake 15-30 minutes depending on how soft you like your cabbage.

> **Frankie's Tip:**
> In choosing mustard, make sure that there is no additional sugar or oil in the mustard. Make sure to read all of the labels of the seasonings used during the protocol from Phase 2. Hidden ingredients could affect your weight loss.

Cole Slaw
1 head of cabbage, shredded
  or the equivalent pre shredded
  packages
1 tsp mustard

5 tbsp Bragg Apple Cider
  Vinegar
½ tsp celery seeds
Pinch of sea salt
Stevia or Xylitol to taste

Whisk all ingredients and pour over cabbage.

> **Frankie's Tip:**
> You may whip ½ cup olive oil into the dressing during Phase 3.

Spinach Chips
1 lb fresh spinach greens   1 lemon, juiced

Place spinach leaves on mesh dehydrator sheets and sprinkle with lemon juice. Dehydrate at 105°F until crunchy. If you don't have a dehydrator, simply put in your oven at the lowest setting for a few hours.

> **Frankie's Tip:**
> These are very tasty with a mixture of lemon juice and salt or chickpea tamari.

Phase 2 Vegetables

Baked Garlic
1 head of garlic or more

Preheat the oven to 400°F. Peel the outer layers of the garlic bulb leaving the skin of the individual cloves intact. Cut off ½ inch of the top of the cloves exposing the individual cloves of garlic. Place the garlic head(s) in a covered baking dish or wrap in aluminum foil. Bake 35-40 minutes. Use a spoon to squeeze out the cooked cloves from the bulbs. Spread on anything! This adds a gourmet touch to any dish.

Frankie's Tip:
For Phase 3 you may drizzle olive oil, macadamia nut oil or coconut oil on the garlic head before you bake it.

Garlic Spinach
1 head of baked garlic
(recipe above)

Spinach (fresh, frozen, baby, cooked or uncooked as long as it is organic)
Sea salt (optional)

Spread the garlic on the steamed or cooked spinach. Add a pinch of sea salt. Terrific!

Frankie's Tip:
Spinach is heavily sprayed with pesticides. It is another one of the dirty dozen vegetables and fruits. Always buy organic.

Radishes!
Once cooked, they lose most of that radish taste.
You can roast them boil them, mash them, grate them.

Phase 2 Meats

Steak & Mustard Sauce
3½ oz steak lean
1 cup beef broth (approx)
  homemade or organic (no oil)

1-2 tbsp sugar-free mustard
½ tsp ground mustard powder
2 tbsp chopped onion

Pour ¼ cup of beef broth and both mustards in a bowl. Mix until smooth. Pour into sauté pan and add steak and onions, coating both with sauce. Cook until steak has reached its desired doneness and add just enough broth to keep the sauce a gravy type consistency. The sauce will thicken a bit more once it cools.

Chili
3½ oz ground steak
1 tomato, ½ diced and ½
  pureed in a food processor
½ cup water or broth
3 cloves garlic, minced
½ tsp onion powder

½ tsp oregano
¼ tsp cumin
¼ tsp black pepper
¼ tsp cayenne
¼ tsp basil
¼ tsp thyme

Preheat skillet over medium heat. Add 1 tbsp of water and the garlic. Sauté 2-3 minutes taking care not to burn the garlic. Add more water or broth as necessary. Increase heat to medium/high and add ground steak – about 5 minutes. Add all of the seasonings and cook an additional 3 minutes. Add more water/broth as necessary. Add tomatoes, tomato puree and balance of the water/broth. Turn heat down to medium-low and simmer until it reaches the desired consistency.

> ### Frankie's Tip:
> Mix all of the spices together in a small bowl so they may be added all at once.

Phase 2 Meats

Beef with Cabbage Lettuce Wraps
3 ½ oz ground beef
1 cup shredded cabbage
2 cloves garlic, minced
2 tbsp fresh cilantro, chopped
¼ cup plus 2 tbsp chicken broth
2 large lettuce leaves
Sea salt (optional) and pepper
  to taste
Hot sauce (optional)

Heat skillet on medium-high. Add ground beef, garlic and 2 tbsp broth. Sauté until almost done. Take out and set aside. Put cabbage in skillet and start to fry to pick up the beef flavor then add the ¼ cup of broth. Cook until tender, not mushy. Add beef and cook for 1 minute on high heat. Add hot sauce if desired. Remove from heat and divide onto lettuce leaves. Wrap up and serve warm.

Steak or Chicken Pizzaiola
3 ½ oz of steak or chicken
1 Tomato, diced
2 cloves of garlic, minced
1 tsp oregano
1 tsp basil
¼ tsp chili powder
Black pepper to taste

Preheat oven to 350°F. Place half of the diced tomatoes in a casserole dish. Layer meat on the tomatoes and sprinkle garlic on top. In a small bowl, toss the rest of the tomato with the oregano, basil, chili powder and pepper. Spoon mixture over steak. Cover tightly with aluminum foil or lid and bake for 45-60 minutes.

Frankie's Tip:
When using chicken, season both sides with salt and pepper and sear until brown before layering on top of the tomatoes.

Phase 2 Meats

Beef Chili

3 ½ oz lean ground beef
1 large tomato
2 cups of water
Season to taste with the
    following spices:

Chili powder
Garlic powder
Black pepper
Cayenne pepper
Sea salt

Grill beef on grill tray, remove all excess fat, then crumble or cut into small pieces. Place beef, tomato, water and seasoning into crock pot for sauce pan. Bring to boil and then turn down heat and simmer for at least 1 hour. Can be stewed in crock pot all day long if desired.

Beef French Dip

3 ½ oz sliced cooked steak
½ onion sliced into rings
1 cup beef broth

2 cloves minced garlic
½ tsp thyme
½ tsp pepper
Bragg Liquid Aminos

Preheat pan over medium heat. Add onions and garlic. Cook 5-10 minutes until tender. Add broth, thyme, and pepper. Bring to boil. Reduce heat and simmer 5-10 minutes. Add steak and return to boil. Reduce heat and simmer 5-10 minutes. Serve steak and onions with the au jus and a couple splashes of liquid aminos.

Crockpot Roast

3 ½ oz steak
Onion soup mix

1 cup beef broth
Black pepper to taste

Add steak to crock pot. Cover with remaining ingredients. Cook for several hours until reaches desired doneness. Serve.

Phase 2 Meats

Down. Set. Chili!
3 ½ oz ground steak
1 tomato
½ cup water or broth
3-4 cloves minced garlic
Seasonings (to taste):
  ½ tsp onion powder

½ tsp oregano
¼ tsp cumin
¼ tsp black pepper
¼ tsp cayenne
¼ tsp basil
¼ tsp thyme

Preheat pan over medium heat. Add minced garlic and 1 tbsp of the water/ broth to pan. Sauté 2-3 mins. Be sure not to burn the garlic. Add more water/broth as necessary. Increase heat to medium-high. Add ground steak and sauté until brown – about 5 minutes. Add all seasonings and cook an additional 3 minutes. Continue to add more water/broth as necessary. While that is cooking dice ½ of tomato and place other ½ in food processor or blender to puree. Mix in tomatoes, puree, and rest of broth. Turn heat down to and simmer until it reaches desired consistency.

TIP: I usually mix all my spices together in a small bowl so I can add them all at once.

Meatballs
3 ½ oz steak
  (ground into hamburger)
1 Grissini (ground into powder)
1 tbsp milk
Parsley

Onion powder
Basil
Oregano
Garlic
Salt
Pepper

Preheat oven to 400°F. In bowl, combine all ingredients. Form into 1" meatballs (makes about 6-7). Place in baking dish or non-stick baking sheet and cook 10 minutes turning halfway through cooking time.

TIP: I usually use a glass baking dish to make these as they seem to want to stick less. Also, if you want to brown them more after cooking, you can grill them for 1-2 mins each side. These also can be frozen in a freezer bag and then warmed up before serving. Makes a great quick meal!

Phase 2 Meats

Meatloaf

3½ oz Ground beef (lean)
for each serving
1 serving Melba toast crumbs
1 ketchup recipe

1 tbsp chopped onion
1 clove minced garlic
Cayenne to taste
¼ tsp paprika

Crush Melba toast into fine powder. Mix with the ground beef, chopped onion and spices. Place in a baking dish, loaf pan or muffin tin for single servings. Baste with ketchup recipe mixture and bake at 350°F for 15-20 minutes. Cook longer for multiple servings using a loaf pan.

Mini-Meat Loaf

3½ oz steak
½ tsp milk or bbq sauce
1 grissini (ground into powder)
2-3 cloves minced garlic
½ tsp dehydrated minced onion
½ tsp spicy mustard

¼ tsp allspice
⅛ tsp sage
Salt/pepper to taste
Any additional seasonings

NOTE: This includes your meat, grissini, and ½ tsp of your daily allowance of milk.

Preheat oven to 350°F. In small bowl combine all ingredients and form into a small meatloaf. Place in glass dish, cover, and bake 25-30 minutes. Uncover dish, add bbq sauce or homemade sugar-free ketchup to top, and bake 5-10 additional minutes. Serve immediately with a bit more of bbq sauce or homemade sugar-free ketchup for dipping.

Ground Beef Tacos

3½ oz lean ground beef
Lettuce leaves
1 tbsp finely minced onion
1 clove crushed & minced garlic
Dash of garlic powder

Dash of onion powder
Dash of dried oregano
Fresh chopped coriander to taste
Cayenne pepper to taste
Salt and black pepper to taste

Brown ground beef. Add onion, garlic, and spices and a little water and simmer gently for 5-10 minutes. Add salt to taste. Serve taco style in butter lettuce or romaine leaf mock tortillas or with a side of tomatoes or salsa.

Phase 2 Shrimp and Fish

Broiled Shrimp
3 ½ oz shrimp
2-3 cup water (enough to cover
  shrimp in pan)

¼ cup apple cider vinegar
2 tbsp seafood seasoning

Add water, apple cider vinegar, seafood seasoning and shrimp to saucepan over medium-high heat. Let water come to slow boil. When shrimp start floating, remove from heat and drain.

Garlic Shrimp
3 ½ oz shrimp
  (peeled & deveined)
4-6 cloves minced garlic or
  1-2 tsp garlic paste

½ cup broth
½ tsp parsley
⅛ tsp dried thyme
⅛ tsp crushed red pepper
1 bay leaf

Heat nonstick pan over medium-high heat. Mix 1 tbsp of the broth with red pepper, minced garlic, and bay leaf. Add to pan. Cook less than a minute. Be sure not to burn the garlic. Add shrimp. Cook 3 minutes. Remove shrimp from pan. Add the remainder of the 1/2 cup broth, parsley, and thyme. Bring to a boil. Cook for 1-2 minutes until reduced by half. Return shrimp to pan and toss to coat. Discard bay leaf and serve.

Prawn Scampi
3 ½ oz grams of prawns
  (peel shell off, weigh out
  3 ½ oz before cooking)
¼ tsp minced Garlic

3 tbsp fresh squeezed
  lemon juice
Dash of onion powder, garlic,
  salt and pepper to taste
¼ cup vegetable broth or water
  (broth gives it more flavor)

In saucepan sauté minced garlic in the lemon juice and vegetable broth. Add dry ingredients. Add prawns and cook till pink or 5-7 minutes.

Phase 2 Shrimp and Fish

Lemon Pepper Fish
3½ oz whitefish
Juice of half lemon
1-3 cloves minced garlic

½ tsp black pepper
¼ tsp salt
¼ tsp cumin powder,
⅛ tsp turmeric

Place fish in small bowl. Add garlic, black pepper, salt, cumin, and turmeric. Ensure to coat both sides. Cover and marinate at least 1 hour in refrigerator. Preheat oven to 400°F. Place the fish in a non-stick baking dish and cover with the marinade. Bake 10-20 minutes depending on thickness, until fish easily flakes. Squeeze with lemon juice.

Shrimp and Asparagus Stir Fry
3½ oz shrimp
(shelled & deveined)

1-2 cloves minced garlic
Asparagus (allowed amount)
1 tbsp fresh ginger

Add shrimp, garlic, and ginger into pre-heated pan. Stir fry for 3-5 minutes. (If needed, add small amount of water.) While that cooks, snap ends off of asparagus. Cut asparagus into 2" pieces. Remove shrimp from pan and add asparagus. Drizzle with a bit of Bragg Liquid Aminos. Stir fry for 2-3 mins. Re-add shrimp to pan and heat for 1 minute to heat through. Serve.

Ginger Mahi Mahi
3½ oz mahi mahi
(or any whitefish)
1 tsp minced garlic

1 tsp ginger black pepper,
(to taste)
Sliced tomato (allowed amount)
Juice of ½ or 1 lemon

Place fish on top of a large sheet non-stick aluminium foil. Cover with garlic, ginger, and pepper. Place tomatoes on top of seasoned fish. Top with squeezed lemon juice. Close up aluminium foil into a "pouch" so that the top and ends are sealed. Bake at 350°F for 10-20 mins. (depending on thickness) or until fish flakes.

Phase 2 Shrimp and Fish

Bake-Ahead Meal Packets

Preparing a few day's worth of these meals is convenient. Many of the vegetables on the diet lend themselves well to the packet cooking method. Using different combinations of vegetables and proteins with different seasoning blends creates variety.

Wash, cut and measure:	3 ½ oz vegetables (spinach,
3 ½ oz lean protein	chard, tomatoes, asparagus,
(chicken, white fish, lobster,	cabbage, cauliflower,
crab, or prawns)	zucchini, fennel/anise)

Assembling the Packets for Cooking: Preheat oven 350°F. Cut pieces of parchment or aluminum foil for the packets (about 14 inches off the roll) Place one serving of vegetables on the parchment/foil. Lightly salt and pepper the vegetables. Place one serving of protein on top of the vegetables. Season with 1 tsp of any sugar-free seasoning blend. Fold parchment/foil to create a packet. Arrange packets on a large cookie/baking sheet and place on the center rack in the oven. Bake for 25 minutes. Allow to rest for 5 minutes and drain off any excess liquid before serving. Dense vegetables, such as fennel and cauliflower, will be crisp-cooked. If softer vegetables are desired, cook packets with these vegetables an additional 5-10 minutes.

Suggested combinations:

Chicken and zucchini with Singapore seasoning

Prawns and tomato with Tandoori seasoning

Tilapia and asparagus with fajita seasoning

Cod and spinach with Italian seasoning

Lobster tail and fennel with seafood seasoning

Phase 2 Shrimp and Fish

Cioppino (Seafood Stew)
3½ oz fish of choice
1 chopped plum tomato
2 cup broth (vegetable or chicken)
1 tsp lemon juice
3 cloves minced garlic
1 bay leaf
1 tsp dehydrated minced onion

1 tsp dried parsley
¼ tsp taragon
¼ tsp basil
⅛ tsp rosemary
⅛ tsp fennel seeds
Dash of Tabasco
Water
Salt and Pepper to taste

In a skillet, put just enough water to cover the fish and poach it until it is cooked through, about 3 minutes. Remove skillet from heat and add the rest of the ingredients. Mix thoroughly and serve.

Frankie's Tip: Chill and serve over a bed of lettuce.

Creole Catfish
(or other white fish)
3½ oz of catfish
1 chopped tomato

½ cup water
1 tsp minced onion
1-2 tsp Cajun seasoning

Preheat skillet over medium-high heat. Place fish, minced onion and Cajun seasoning in a Ziploc bag and shake to coat fish. Add water to skillet and poach fish 3-4 minutes. Add more water if skillet becomes dry. Add tomatoes and poach for 5-10 minutes until tomatoes are tender and sauce is a soupy consistency.

Curried Broiled Fish
3½ oz of fish of choice
1 sliced tomato

½ lemon
1 tsp curry seasoning

Preheat broiler. Place fish on boiler pan, squeeze lemon over fish and sprinkle with curry. Place tomatoes on top of fish. Broil 8-10" away from broiler for 10-15 minutes until tomato starts to blacken. Serve.

Frankie's Tip:
It is also great on the grill. This dish includes both your protein and vegetable in one meal.

Phase 2 Shrimp and Fish

Curried Prawns

3 ½ oz prawns
1 onion, chopped
1 tsp garlic paste or
   3 cloves minced

⅛ cup of water
½ tsp curry powder
¼ tsp cumin
Sea salt (optional) and pepper
   to taste

Preheat skillet over medium-high. Add water and cook onion and garlic until tender. Add prawns and seasonings. Stir and cook until the prawns are cooked through. Serve.

Faux Prawn Fried Rice

3 ½ oz prawns
3-4 cups shredded cabbage
4 tsp chicken or vegetable broth
½ tsp onion powder
½ tsp garlic powder OR
  1 clove fresh garlic, minced

1 ½ tsp Bragg Liquid Aminos
Black pepper to taste
Red pepper flakes to taste
  (optional)

Preheat skillet over medium-high heat. Add cabbage, 2 tbsp of broth and ½ tsp Bragg Liquid Aminos to pan. Stir fry until the cabbage is tender. Remove the cabbage and place on serving dish. Sprinkle with black pepper. Turn heat down to medium. Add prawns, 2 tbsp of broth, onion powder, garlic and 1 tsp Bragg Liquid Aminos. Stir fry until prawns are pink. Sprinkle red pepper flakes (optional). Serve immediately over cabbage.

Frankie's Tip:

You may alter the amount of water and Bragg Liquid Amino to taste. You may also substitute water for broth. Don't expect the cabbage to taste like rice but it is soft and crunchy at the same time and goes really well with the prawns.

Phase 2 Shrimp and Fish

Fish Tacos
3 ½ oz white fish
1 garlic clove, minced
¼ cup chopped onion
1 chopped tomato or
 ¼ cup salsa

Squeeze of lime juice
2 tbsp cilantro, chopped
Sea salt and pepper to taste
Lettuce leaves
 (butter lettuce or your choice)
Shredded cabbage (optional)

Sauté fish with onion and garlic in a little water. Break apart fish while cooking. When fish is cooked through, squeeze on lime juice, season with salt (optional) and pepper. Spread on lettuce leaves and top with cilantro, tomatoes and optional cabbage. Roll into a wrap and serve.

Phase 2 Chicken

Chicken Chili
3 ½ oz chicken breast
1 cup chopped tomatoes
 (I removed the skin)
1 ½ cup of water
1 tbsp apple cider vinegar
Onion powder to taste
3 cloves of garlic, minced

1 tsp garlic powder
2 tsp of chili powder
 (or to taste) - DIVIDED
2 large dashes of Hot Sauce
 - DIVIDED
Dash of cayenne pepper
Salt and pepper to taste

In one saucepan put 1 cup of water, 1 tbsp of chili powder, 1 tsp of garlic powder, large dash of hot sauce, salt and pepper, bring to boil and add chicken. Once chicken is done take out to cool and shred. In another saucepan, I use the smallest one, I have put in 1 cup of tomatoes, 1 tbsp apple cider vinegar, onion powder, minced garlic, 1 tbsp of chili powder, large dash of hot sauce, and salt and pepper to taste, bring to a boil to cook tomatoes down. You might need to add more seasoning to taste or water to get to the consistency you desire once the tomatoes are cooked down add the shredded chicken and let simmer.

This had lots of flavor and I really enjoyed the sauce, it even thickened some and was dark brown like chili sauce would be. Served with a Grissini bread stick.

Phase 2 Chicken

Chicken Gravy   1 grissini
½ cup chicken broth
  (home made is better)

Add ¼ cup broth to small saucepan and bring to boil. While broth is heating, grind grissini in food processor until it is a powder. (I use my coffee grinder.) Add the powdered grissini to the pan, whisking constantly until dissolved. Still whisking, add remaining ¼ cup broth. Reduce heat to medium and whisk for 3-4 minutes, until thickened. I usually add some salt, pepper, thyme, sage, or poultry seasoning, etc for more flavor. Feel free to add any spices you like.

TIP: I pour this over my boiled chicken that I use to make my broth. This gives it a lot more flavor as boiled chicken is usually pretty bland.

Chicken Marinara   1 tsp oregano
3½ oz chicken   1 tsp basil
1 small tomato, diced   ½ tsp chili powder
2-3 cloves of garlic   A dash of garlic powder
                                    A dash of pepper

Preheat oven to 350°F. Place ½ of the diced tomatoes in a casserole dish. Sear chicken on both sides for 1 to 2 minutes per side with a dash of garlic powder, salt and pepper in the pan as it cooks. Place the seared chicken on top of the tomatoes in the casserole dish with the minced garlic. In a small bowl, toss the remaining diced tomatoes with the remaining seasonings. Place the contents of the bowl on top of the chicken. Cover the dish tightly with foil (or use the lid if you have one). Cook for 45-60 minutes and serve warm.

Chicken Wrap   ½ cup onion
3½ oz chicken breast   ½ cup diced tomato
Dash of salt, pepper and   2 tbsp chopped coriander
  garlic powder   1 head lettuce

Season chicken breast with salt, pepper and garlic powder on George Foreman grill. Once done (3 to 4 minutes) cut into strips or shred. Sauté onions in a separate pan using small dab of organic coconut oil. Clean lettuce and pat dry. Place chicken breast on lettuce, add onions and tomatoes and wrap. You can add additional shredded lettuce.

Phase 2 Chicken

Faux Bruschetta
3 ½ oz chicken diced
2 ½ oz cherry tomato's halved
3 large leaves of basil,
    julienned or chopped
2 tbsp water
4 drops liquid lemon Stevia
    (may omit)
1-2 tsp balsamic vinegar or
    apple cider
Garlic salt, lemon pepper,
    salt to taste

In small skillet heat water, add chicken and spices, cook until chicken begins to turn white, add one half the basil, sauté just a minute until chicken done. Add tomato's remaining basil and sauté a couple minutes until water is evaporated. Get pan really hot, move ingredients to side of pan, add balsamic then mix in chicken mixture. Voila' Yum Yum!! I ate it just like this but you could put on melba toast.

Grilled Chicken Salad
3 ½ oz of chicken breast
¼ tsp garlic
Dash of Sweet basil
Dash of thyme
Dash of onion powder
Dash of salt & pepper to taste
Spinach

Season both sides of chicken breast with seasoning above. On George Foreman grill chicken for 3-4 minutes (depending on thickness of chicken but do cook till done.) While that is cooking prep spinach. Rinse and dry, place in bowl. Once chicken is done cut into cubes on a plate. Scrape juice and cubes into bowel of spinach. The natural juice from the chicken should be enough to not need any dressing.

Asian Ginger Chicken
3 ½ oz chicken
¼ cup organic chicken broth
    or water
4 tbsp lemon juice
¼ tsp lemon or orange zest
½ tsp fresh ginger
4 tsp Bragg's Liquid Aminos
1 tsp chopped onion
Stevia to taste
Salt and pepper to taste
Cayenne pepper to taste

In a small sauce pan, sauté chicken in a little lemon juice and water until slightly browned. Add spices, ginger, salt, lemon and Stevia. Add Bragg's liquid aminos and cook thoroughly. Deglaze the pan periodically by adding a little water. Serve hot and garnish with lemon or orange slices.

Phase 2 Chicken

Sweet N Spicy Chicken Wraps
3 ½ oz chicken
4 cabbage leaves, whole
1 gala apple, small, cored
   and chopped
2 tbsp Bragg Liquid Aminos
Water

1 tbsp Tabasco
1 tbsp mustard, course, ground
2 cloves of garlic, minced
2 tsp chicken or beef broth
1 tsp onion powder
1 tsp garlic powder
Pepper to taste

In a small skillet sauté chicken with Bragg's Liquid Aminos, pepper, onion powder and garlic powder. Cook until done, adding water to periodically deglaze the pan and keep the chicken moist. In a large high sided pan boil the cabbage leaves one at a time until tender and pliable. As they are done, set aside to cool. When the chicken is done (leaving the juices in the pan), remove and set aside to cool, and then chop into small pieces. Add the garlic, mustard and broth to the juices in the pan, bring to a boil and add the apple. Once the apple starts to become tender add back the chicken and Tabasco. Spread mixture on cabbage leaves and roll up.

Phase 2 Vegetarian

Frankie's Tip

As a vegetarian I choose not to eat meat, chicken or fish yet I have had much success on the hCG protocol. My protein sources comes from eggs, egg whites, skim milk cottage cheese and whey protein (good, clean no additives).

My typical phase 2 day will include:

Breakfast
Coffee with organic soy creamer, almond, hemp or coconut milk

Lunch
3½ oz of skim milk cottage cheese, grilled asparagus

Dinner
1 organic egg and 3 egg whites baked with onions

Snacks
Apple, grapefruit

Make sure you always choose organic apples; they are another on the dirty dozen list.

Asparagus Frittata
3 egg whites
1 whole egg
Asparagus (allowed amount)
1-2 cloves minced garlic

1 tbsp dehydrated minced
 Onion
1 tbsp water
1 tsp parsley
Salt/pepper (to taste)
Tabasco (optional)

Preheat pan over medium heat. Snap woody ends off asparagus and discard. Snap each asparagus spear into 2-3 pieces. Add to pan with garlic and heat through until tender. Preheat oven to 400°F. In bowl, mix eggs and water. Add asparagus, minced onion, parsley, salt/pepper. Pour egg mixture into non-stick baking dish (or dish lined with parchment paper). Place in oven and cook 10-15 minutes until done. Top with Tabasco (optional) and serve immediately.

Phase 2 Vegetarian

Eggs with Vegetable(s)

1 organic egg

3 eggs whites

Choice of one per meal:
  chopped spinach, garlic,

organic tomatoes, grilled
asparagus, onions baked
in the oven until wilted.

Sea Salt (optional)

Whip the egg and eggs whites with a little water, add one vegetable. Pan fry or broil until the eggs puff up. Sprinkle with sea salt (optional).

Cilantro Cottage Cheese
Stuffed Pepper

½ cup cottage cheese

1 pepper of your choice, yellow,
  red or green

1 tsp cilantro

1 tsp chives

Sea salt to taste

Preheat oven to 350°F. Clean out a pepper and roast it in the oven until soft. In a bowl, combine the cottage cheese and all of the spices. Stuff the pepper with the mixture and bake it in the oven until it bubbles or eat as is.

Stuffed Egg Salad in Tomatoes

1 whole hardboiled egg

3 hardboiled egg whites

1 large heirloom or very ripe
  tomato

Pinch of sea salt to taste

¼ cup apple cider vinegar

1 tsp Stevia or Xylitol

1 tsp mustard (optional)

1 tsp chives

Chop the eggs with the vinegar and combine with all of the spices. Slice the tomato in half and take out seeds. Stuff the mixture into the tomato halves.

Egg White Soufflé

1 whole egg

3 egg whites

1 tbsp milk or soy milk

Sea salt and pepper to taste

¼ tsp garlic powder

¼ tsp onion powder

In a bowl, beat the eggs with a mixer and all of the spices. Pour into the pie plate and broil until the eggs fluff up like a soufflé. Serve with a side of broiled asparagus sprinkled with lemon juice and sea salt for a complete meal.

Phase 2 Vegetarian

Grilled Tofu Spinach
4 oz of firm tofu marinated in
   homemade ketchup
   (use our recipe)

1 package of fresh or frozen
   organic spinach
1 clove of garlic, minced

Preheat the oven to 350°F. Sauté the garlic and spinach until the spinach is wilted. Place the spinach in the baking dish as the bottom layer and top with the tofu. Bake for 10 minutes.

Ginger Spinach Tofu
4 oz firm organic tofu,
   cut in cubes
1 tbsp ginger, freshly grated

1 package of fresh or frozen
   organic spinach
¼ cup vinegar
½ tsp Xylitol or Stevia
¼ tsp nutmeg

Preheat oven to 350°F. In a bowl, combine all of the ingredients. Bake for 10 minutes. Alternately, you may sauté this in a pan.

Tomato Basil Salad
4 oz of firm tofu, cubed
1 large tomato, cut up
1 yellow onion, sliced

¼ cup chopped basil
¼ cup vinegar
1 tsp Xylitol
Pinch of seas salt and pepper

Mix all of the ingredients together and allow to marinate in the refrigerator for a few hours. Great on a hot day.

> **Frankie's Tip:**
> Ordinarily I don't like to mix two vegetables but I make an exception with the onions and tomatoes.

Phase 2 Vegetarian

Fennel Salad

1 bulb of fennel with fronds, chopped medium in a food processor

1 scoop of protein powder

2 tbsp spicy mustard

1 tbsp brown rice vinegar

½ tsp sea salt

⅛ tsp cayenne pepper

¼ cup lemon juice

¼ cup water

Konjac flour noodles (optional)

In a blender, blend mustard, vinegar, salt, pepper, protein and lemon with the water until it becomes a sauce. Toss sauces with the fennel and optional Konjac flour noodles (for bulk).

Apple Tofu Salad

4 oz tofu, cubed

1 cucumber

½ apple

¼ cup vinegar

¼ tsp sea salt

1 tsp Xylitol

Mix all of the ingredients together and allow to marinate in the refrigerator for a few hours.

Vanilla Protein Drink

1 scoop of hemp powder

¾ cup of water

1 tbsp milk or soy milk

1 tbsp vanilla

Xylitol or Stevia to taste

Blend it all together. Organic strawberries may also be added for a refreshing delight in the Spring and Summer.

Frankie's Tip:

Certified organic hemp protein powder is one of the most powerful forms of protein. As a vegetarian, it is important that you have clean protein. When I do the protocol I add whey protein and organic hemp a few times a week making sure the protein powders are clean, with no added sugars. On a busy day, I travel with my protein drink and have a cucumber salad on the side.

Phase 2 Vegetarian

Chocolate Pudding Tofu for
Lunch (Yes, for lunch)
2 scoops of CocoPure Tea

4 oz of tofu
2 packets of Xylitol
1 tsp vanilla

Put all of the ingredients in a Vit-a-Blend or other blender and blend until smooth. With a side of greens this is a complete lunch.

Coffee Tofu Ice Cream
(Another lunch)
1 tbsp milk or soy milk
4 oz tofu, soft

¾ cup coffee (can be cold)
2-3 tsp of Xylitol to taste
1/2 cup ice cubes
1 tbsp vanilla

Put all of the ingredients in the Vit-a-Mix and blend. Add ice cubes and blend until thick like an ice cream. Add more sweetener if desired.

Apple Pudding
1 granny smith apple, peeled
   and cut in half
1 scoop of whey powder
¼ pkg Konjac flour noodles,
   long ones cut up, or vegan
   shrimp

1 cup water
Stevia to taste
¼ tsp cinnamon (optional)
⅛ tsp ginger powder
   (optional)

In a blender, puree ½ of the apple, whey powder, water, cinnamon, Stevia and ginger. Chopped the remaining ½ apple. Pour mixture over the noodles and chopped apple.

> **Frankie's Tip:**
> Substitute ¼ cup of strawberries for the apple and you have strawberry pudding.

Phase 2 Vegetarian

Cucumber Apple Slaw
1 cucumber
1 small apple
½ small lemon
1 scoop of protein powder
Stevia to taste

¼ tsp garlic powder
Dash of mustard powder
Dash of cinnamon, sea salt and
   white or cayenne pepper
½ bag of Konjac flour noodles
(optional)

In a food processor, blend all ingredients except the noodles until cucumber is chopped appealingly. Serve atop noodles.

> **Frankie's Tip:**
> Konjac flour noodles have no calories and are can be very creative to cook with.

Fennel Salad
1 bulb of fennel with fronds,
   chopped medium in a food
   processor
1 scoop of protein powder
2 tbsp spicy mustard

1 tbsp brown rice vinegar
½ tsp sea salt
⅛ tsp cayenne pepper
¼ cup lemon juice
¼ cup water
Konjac flour noodles (optional)

In a blender, blend mustard, vinegar, salt, pepper, protein and lemon with the water until it becomes a sauce. Toss sauces with the fennel and optional Konjac flour noodles (for bulk).

Phase 3 Recipes

Make sure to weigh yourself every day on Phase 3. You may be sensitive to some of these products and gain a pound or two. What may work for me may make you gain weight and the reverse is also true. One of my favorite books for gluten free recipes is *The Gluten-Free Almond Flour Cookbook*.

Some of my resources for gluten free baking come from several books. I can recommend these two: *The Gluten Free Almond Flour Cookbook* by Elana Amsterdam found at www.elanaspantry.com and *Gluten Free Recipes for the Conscious Cook, A Seasonal Vegetarian Cookbook* by Leslie Cerier found at www.lesliecerier.com

Dressings, Seasonings & Sauces

Cucumber Sauce
2 tbsp fat free cottage cheese
½ of a peeled/seeded
   cucumber cut into chunks
1 tsp garlic
¼ tsp onion powder
Touch of salt/pepper

Mix all ingredients in blender. Refrigerate until cold, serve.

Mayonnaise Dressing
⅛ tsp paprika
1 cup olive oil
¼ tsp salt
1 tbsp lemon juice
1 egg yolk
1 tbsp vinegar

Mix the salt and pepper and add the egg yolk. Beat until thickened a little; gradually add the lemon juice and vinegar. Using an egg beater, beat in the oil, one tsp at a time. Beat thoroughly after each addition of oil. Cover the dressing with an earthen or glass dish and let stand in a cool place until ready to use. Half this quantity of dressing may be made by dividing the yolk of egg. In making this dressing, all of the acid must be added to the yolk before beginning with the oil.

Phase 3 Vegetables

How to Cook Spaghetti Squash

Bake it:
Preheat the oven to 375°F. Pierce the whole shell several times with a fork or skewer. Place in baking dish. Bake in oven for approximately 1 hour until flesh is tender.

Boil it:
Heat a pot of water large enough to hold the whole squash. Place the entire squash into the boiling water and cook for 20-30 minutes depending on its size. It is done when a fork goes into the flesh easily.

Microwave it:
Cut squash in half lengthwise; remove seeds. Place squash, cut sides up, in a microwave dish with ¼ cup of water. Cover with plastic wrap and cook on high for 10-12 minutes, depending on size of squash. Add more cooking time if necessary. Let stand covered for 5 minutes. With fork "comb" out the strands.

Slow Cooker or Crock Pot:
Choose a smaller spaghetti squash (unless you have an extra large slow cooker) so that it will fit. Add 2 cups of water to the slow cooker. Pierce the whole shell with a large fork or skewer, add to crock pot, cover and cook on low 8-9 hours. Once the squash is cooked, let it cool for 10-20 minutes so it will be easier to handle. Cut in half and remove the seeds. Pull a fork lengthwise through the flesh to separate into long strands. You can cook the spaghetti squash ahead of time and then prepare your favorite recipe.

Phase 3 Vegetables

Spaghetti Squash with Mozzarella

1 spaghetti squash cooked by
   your favorite method and
   separated into strands

1 tbsp Olive oil
¾ cup pesto sauce of your choice
4 oz smoked or plain
   mozzarella cheese, shredded
¼ cup grated Parmesan cheese

Heat oil in large skillet over medium high heat. Add spaghetti squash. Using 2 forks to lift, mix in pesto. Cook just long enough to heat through, mix in cheeses. Heat until everything is well mixed and cheese is beginning to melt. Serve immediately.

> **Frankie's Tip:**
> Spaghetti squash is one of my favorite vegetables. It is much underrated and yet there are so many delicious ways to make it including sweet and savory dishes.

Baked Tomatoes and Cheese Spaghetti Squash

1 spaghetti squash cooked by
   your favorite method and
   separated into strands

½ - 1 cup of marinara sauce
¼ cup quality grated cheese
½ cup Ricotta cheese
Pinch of sea salt (optional)

Preheat oven to 350°F. In a large bowl toss the squash with the marinara sauce, ricotta cheese and sea salt. Place in a baking dish and sprinkle the grated cheese on top. Bake approximately 5 minutes until the cheese melts.

Melty Cheese, Squash and Chickpea Delight

8 cups diced zucchini, Zephyr
   or summer squash
¼ cup Pecorino Romano
4 cup diced tomatoes,
   or 4 cup tomato sauce
6-8 cloves finely minced garlic
4 cup cooked chickpeas
   (drained), or 2 cans Eden

1 tsp dried oregano
6 cup shredded cheese* such as
   Monterey Jack
1 tsp dried basil
1 tsp dried thyme
4 cup shredded cheese*
   for topping
¼ cup extra virgin olive oil
cheddar, Asiago, havarti or leftover bits of any cheese you have to use up.

Mix ingredients together and bake at 350°F for 30-45 minutes. Serves 8

Phase 3 Vegetables

Raisin Sweet Spaghetti
Squash
1 spaghetti squash cooked by
  your favorite method and
  separated into strands
¼ cup raisins
½ cup ricotta cheese

1 egg
1 tbsp cinnamon
½ tsp vanilla
¼ cup Oh Agave, Xylitol
  or Stevia to taste
Coconut or olive oil spray
Yogurt (optional)

Preheat oven to 350°F. Beat the egg, cheese, raisins, cinnamon, vanilla and Oh Agave together. In a large bowl, toss the wet ingredients with the squash. Grease a large baking dish with either coconut or olive oil spray. Transfer the squash to the baking dish and bake for 25 minutes. Serve warm with yogurt.

Gluten-Free Salt and Vinegar
Kale Chips
1 head of kale, red or green,
  chopped into chip size pieces

1 tsp olive oil or coconut oil
1 tbsp apple cider vinegar
1 tsp sea salt

Preheat oven to 375°F. Place kale in a large bowl. Drizzle with oil & vinegar, then sprinkle with salt. Massage in with your hands. Line 2 baking sheets with parchment paper. Spread out the kale so that pieces do not touch. Bake for 10-13 minutes until dry and crispy. Cool 10 minutes and serve.

Cauliflower Red Onion Baked
Delight
1 head of cauliflower, cut up
1 small red onion

2 tbsp coconut oil
½ cup good Italian Parmesan
  cheese, grated
1 tsp sea salt

Preheat oven to 350°F. Spray a casserole dish with the oil spray and bake the onions in it, covered, until they are wilted. Add the cauliflower, salt and spread the coconut oil on top. Cover and bake for 30-35 minutes. Right before serving, sprinkle the grated cheese on top and place under broiler for 5 minutes.

Frankie's Tip:
As a vegetarian, I use a lot of coconut products for Phase 3 including: coconut oil, coconut flour, coconut palm sugar and coconut milk products.

Phase 3 Vegetables

Crispy Spinach   ¼ cup sesame or coconut oil
1 package of fresh spinach   Pinch of sea salt

Preheat oven to 400°F. In a large bowl toss the spinach with the oil and salt. Spread on a baking sheet and bake for 10 minutes until crispy. Alternately the spinach may be cooked in a wok, being tossed continuously until crispy.

Creamed Spinach   ¾ tsp garlic chopped
1 package of fresh spinach   1 tsp + pinch cayenne
¾ stick butter   Tarragon, nutmeg, garlic
1 qt heavy cream   to taste

Warm butter over medium-high. Add chopped garlic, sauté. Add heavy cream. Blend on medium-high whisk until blended. Turn to medium-low when it gets foamy and cook until thick. Add spices. Then add spinach and turn in cream until bright green (do not overcook).

Mashed Cauliflower   2 tbsp organic butter or coconut
2 heads of cauliflower, washed   oil or 1 tbsp each
  and cut into large pieces   ½ tsp sea salt

Preheat oven to 350°F. Steam cauliflower until very tender. Either puree cauliflower in a food processor or mash with a fork. Mix in butter and/or coconut oil and salt. Bake in a casserole dish for 20 minutes. Serve warm.

Sweet Potato & Carrot Oven Fries   2 tbsp olive oil or coconut oil
6 lg carrots or sweet potatoes   ½ tsp sea salt

Preheat oven to 425°F. Cut up carrots or sweet potatoes (leaving skins on) into sticks. In a large bowl toss with olive oil and salt. Line a baking sheet with parchment paper. Spread out sticks on baking sheet and bake 18-22 minutes until browned.

Caramelized Onions
Cut 1 large onion into large rough onions or chucks, separating layers. Put on medium heat with some high temp oil (macadamia nut, coconut or butter) Add 1 rounded tbsp Dandy Blend (per onion). Simmer covered for 5-7 minutes, stirring only to keep the onion from sticking.

Phase 3 Vegetables

Portobello Mushrooms
Drench with olive oil and minced garlic. Place on grill cap side down,
then turn and add Parmesan on top.

Phase 3 Pizza

Craving Pizza? Legal Phase 3
Pizza. So good and easy!

2 cups almond flour
1 tsp Celtic sea salt
1 tsp baking soda

½ cup Parmesan cheese
½ cup low fat grated cheese
1 organic egg
1 cup tomato sauce
Vegetable toppings of your
  choice

Preheat oven to 375°F. In a large bowl combine almond flour, Parmesan
cheese, salt and baking soda. In a small bowl, whisk the egg. Mix wet
ingredients with the dry and knead with your hands into a firm dough ball
2/3 inch thick. Place on a pan and bake for 9-10 minutes. When you take it
out of the oven, top with tomato sauce, grated cheese, vegetables and onions
of your choice. Place under broiler to melt the cheese.

Variations:
Pizza is such a versatile dish. There are many ways to create it using
different ingredients. I have tried, and loved adding ½ cup chopped
onions to the dough itself. I also added fresh garlic, 1 tsp of chili
powder or ½ cup sun dried tomatoes. A few sprigs of rosemary or
¼ cup sesame seeds either sprinkled on top or in the dough. Be creative and try all or some of these variations with this basic recipe. For
bite sized pieces, cut the dough into triangles with a metal spatula and
place it on a parchment paper lined baking sheet before baking.

Frankie's Tip:
Many places sell almond flour, yes it's just finely ground almonds,
gluten free. I find the best and least expensive to be sold at Trader
Joe's, referred to as Almond Meal. When possible, buy aluminum
free baking soda and powder as well as alcohol free vanilla. This
is another way to lessen the number of toxins we consume.

Phase 3 Vegetarian

Deviled Eggs
4 hardboiled eggs
Minced tomato
Minced fresh parsley

Salt and pepper to taste
Cut eggs in half and throw out
3 of the 4 yolks.

Mince tomato and parsley. Mix in with the final yolk. Adding salt and pepper. Add a tiny splash of apple cider vinegar. Fill the egg whites (not enough to actually "mound" the whites, but plenty for each).

Herbed Omelet
Makes Multiple Servings
$\frac{1}{8}$ - $\frac{1}{4}$ organic chicken broth
$\frac{1}{4}$ cup(s) pepper(s), red, bell, diced
$\frac{1}{4}$ cup(s) scallion(s) (green onions), sliced
1 clove(s) garlic, minced
10 slice(s) Melba Toast, whole-wheat

$\frac{1}{4}$ cup(s) cottage cheese, low fat
3 egg(s)
8 egg white(s)
$\frac{3}{4}$ cup(s) milk, fat-free evaporated
1 tbsp basil, fresh, minced
1 tbsp rosemary, fresh, minced
2 tsp chives, fresh, minced
1 tbsp parsley, fresh, minced

Preheat the oven to 350°F. Sauté the pepper, and scallions in chicken broth for 6 minutes. Add the garlic and sauté for 3 more minutes. Place the toast slices in a large casserole dish. Combine the remaining ingredients and pour the egg mixture on top of the toast. Add the cooked vegetables. Bake for about 25-40 minutes until the omelet is slightly puffed and set.

Phase 3 Vegetarian

Quiche
5 eggs
2 cups half and half
⅛ tsp nutmeg
1 tsp basil
Hint of cayenne
1 cup diced chunks mozzarella

⅔ cup goat cheese
½ cup shredded Parmesan
   cheese
1 cup diced tomatoes, peppers,
   onions, mushrooms
You can also added prosciutto.
7 oz fresh spinach

Pour egg mixture over baked crust. Bake at 350°F for 45 min. Add shredded cheese and bake 15 more minutes. Let cool a few minutes before serving.

Quiche Crust
½ cup coconut flour
½ cup hazelnut flour
¼ tsp onion salt

¼ cup melted butter
1 egg
1 tbsp Salba
1 tbsp rosemary
   (or whatever spice you want)

Pat into quiche dish. Bake at 400°F for about 15 minutes.

Phase 3 Vegetarian Seafood

Sushi
3 tbsp ground chia seeds in
  2 tbsp water to make a paste
1 heaping tbsp roasted sesame
  seeds (optional) – (Doesn't
  matter if they are ground.)
¾ cup hemp seeds

Cut ¼ cup raw red peppers
  (I used about ½ of a pepper)
¼ cup avocado
  (I used about ½ of the Avacado)
¼ cup Jicama (about the same
  amount as the peppers)
Nori seaweed sheets

Mix together first three ingredients and add a little All Natural Bragg Liquid Aminos all purpose seasoning (to taste... just a small amount). Spread the hemp seed mixture over the seaweed, leaving the bottom row without the hemp seed mixture. Put the peppers, avocado, and jicama on the end of the roll, and roll it all up. Dip in the wasabi, then cover with a slice of pickled ginger. Dip the other side in Bragg's Liquid Amino seasoning.

Phase 3 Chicken

Val's Crunchy Parmesan Chicken Tenders
Olive oil cooking spray
1 cup egg whites
1½ pounds chicken tenders (about 18)
½ tsp sea salt
Freshly ground black pepper
1¼ cups freshly grated Parmesan
¾ cups Italian-style seasoned bread crumbs

Preheat the oven to 475°F. Place the grated Parmesan in a separate dish, and your egg whites in another. Dip the chicken tenders in the egg whites, making sure to coat them thoroughly. Remove the chicken tenders from the egg whites and dredge them in the grated Parmesan to coat completely, pressing to adhere. Spray a large heavy sauté pan with cooking spray and brown the coated chicken tenders 2-3 minutes on each side, on medium-high heat. After your tenders have browned, place the sauté pan in the oven on 475°F for about 10 minutes – or until fully cooked. Transfer the chicken tenders to a platter and serve.

Breadless Burgers
2 large tomatoes, dice
½ red onion, diced
2 tbsp red wine vinegar
Tbsp olive oil
½ tsp oregano
½ tsp basil
Salt and pepper to taste

4 Hamburger Patties (Beef, Turkey or Buffalo)
Grated Parmesan or crumbled Bleu cheese

Combine tomatoes, onions, vinegar, olive oil, oregano, basil, salt and pepper. Stir well then set aside. Grill or fry patties. While patties cook place the cheese on plates (in a flattened pile not much bigger than the patties are round) then place hot cooked patties on top of cheese and top with the tomato onion mixture. Serve.

The reason for using either Parmesan or Bleu cheese is because they don't really melt. If you were to use cheddar or mozzarella it would melt and become a huge mess.

Phase 3 Konjac Flour Noodles Recipes

Chinese Coleslaw with Konjac flour noodles

2-3 bags of Konjac flour noodles pasta
3 tbsp hoisin sauce
2 tbsp red wine vinegar
1 tbsp fresh lime juice
1 tbsp sesame oil
1 tsp Xylitol
2 cups packed Mesclun (2 oz) - also called Field Greens or Spring Mix, is a classic green salad mix
1½ cups finely shredded red cabbage
1½ cups finely shredded green cabbage
1 large celery rib, cut into 2-inch julienned strips
1 small carrot, cut into 2 inch julienned strips
1 scallion, cut into 2 inch julienned strips
One 2 oz piece of jicama, peeled and cut into 2 inch julienned strips (½ cup)
⅓ seedless cucumber, peeled and cut into 2 inch julienned strips (½ cup)
1 tbsp chopped cilantro
2 tbsp thinly sliced basil leaves

You can add your favorite protein: grilled shrimp, chicken, fish, etc., or eat as is.

Empty Konjac flour noodles into a colander draining the water that the noodles are packed in. Boil for one minute, drain in colander and squeeze dry with a small hand towel. Cut noodles into smaller pieces with a scissors. Set aside and let cool.

In a small bowl, whisk the hoisin sauce with the vinegar, lime juice, sesame oil and sugar, stirring to dissolve the sugar.

In a large bowl, toss the mesclun with the red and green cabbages, celery, carrot, scallion, jicama, cucumber, snow peas, and cilantro. Add the dressing and Konjac flour noodles and toss to coat. Garnish with fresh basil.

Serves 8

Phase 3 Konjac Flour Noodles Recipes

Lemon Garlic Konjac flour noodles
3 bags of Konjac flour noodles
⅓ cup of fresh lemon juice
2 tsp fresh minced garlic
½ tsp sea salt
2 tsp sugar
½ tsp mild dijon mustard
1 ½ tbsp extra virgin olive oil
¼ cup toasted pine nuts
¼ cup fresh parsley chopped

Using a whisk, combine lemon juice, garlic, salt, sugar, mustard and olive oil (starting with 1 tbsp) in a bowl.

Drain noodles in colander and rinse well with fresh water. Empty contents of noodles into colander, draining the water that the noodles are packed in. Boil the noodles for one minute, drain in colander, pat dry with a small hand towel and return to pot.

Toss with lemon dressing, toasted nuts and parsley. Season to taste, adding extra olive oil and salt and pepper, if desired. Grate a small amount of Parmesan cheese on top of the noodles (optional).

Ramen dish / Miso
Ramen is a stock made from meat or fish bones flavored with soy, ginger, garlic & Kombu (dried kelp)
Konjac flour noodles 8 oz per person
Rahmen stock or Miso
2 tbsp spring onion
¼ cup bean sprouts/ shoots
3 ½ oz poached or roasted chicken
3 ½ oz roast BBQ pork
Broccoli 2 flowers
¼ zucchini
3 Snow peas
¼ Bok Choy
1 tsp Benito Flakes

Pre cook the noodles in boiling water, place the cooked vegetables in bowl with noodles add pork and chicken then pour boiling stock over the top garnish with spring onions and bonito flakes.

Phase 3 Konjac Flour Noodles Recipes

Singapore Seafood Stir Fry
1 egg beaten
Veggies of choice
(carrot, capsicum, onion etc.)

Konjac flour noodles
1 tsp curry powder
1 tsp crushed garlic
Prawns 4-5 per person
Squid 5 small pieces each

Heat wok, coat with a little oil. Add beaten egg, then vegetables, and garlic. Reheat precooked seafood and noodles in boiling water. Add curry powder to the wok. Season with salt and serve.

Thai Chicken and Noodle Salad (serves 3-4)
Konjac flour noodles
Poached chicken in master
  stock 4 oz shredded
¼ cup red cabbage
¼ cup bean shoots
¼ cup iceberg lettuce
Coriander pinch of leaves
Thai basil pinch

Mint pinch
1 tbsp spring onion
2 tbsp red onion
2 tsp peanuts (optional)
1 tsp black sesame seeds
Thai chili and lime dressing
Sweet chili sauce
Fresh lime juice
White vinegar
Fish sauce

Precook and refresh the Konjac flour noodles. Combine all other ingredients in a large bowl and dress with the Thai dressing.

Phase 3 Desserts and Treats

Gluten-Free Scones

2 cup almond flour
¾ tsp baking soda, aluminum free
½ cup organic raisins
¼ cup pecans or nut of your choice (optional)
1 tsp orange zest (optional)
1 egg
3 tbsp Oh Agave nectar

Preheat oven to 350°F. In a large bowl combine almond flour, baking soda and raisins. In a smaller bowl combine egg and agave nectar. Mix wet ingredients into dry. Knead dough to incorporate ingredients and form into a flat circle. Cut into 8 slices like a pizza and bake for 10-15 minutes.

> ## Frankie's Tip:
> Almond flour can be used in savory recipes or a substitute for most flours in baking. I recommend a few sweeteners, one that is the lowest glycemic index is a brand called Oh Agave. I also use palm sugar (also called coconut sugar), Xylitol, Stevia and sometimes a combination of them.

Mounds Candy

¼ cup sugar-free dark chocolate
1 tbsp Oh Agave
½ cup shredded unsweetened coconut

Melt chocolate in a small pan over very low heat. Using a pastry brush, paint the sides and bottom of a candy mold and place in freezer for 10 minutes until the chocolate hardens. In a small bowl combine the shredded coconut with the Oh Agave. Remove the molds from the freezer and fill the molds with the coconut mixture. Paint chocolate over the coconut mixture to cover the bars. Place back in the freezer for 10 minutes. Turn the hardened mold upside down and pop out the candy. Warning! Try to eat just one.

Almond Cashew Protein Ice Cream – for lunch!

½ cup almond and cashew unsweetened cream (made by Minicreme)
1 heaping tbsp of vanilla whey protein or 1 tbsp of hemp protein
1 tsp vanilla
½ cup ice

Mix the liquid in blender. Add ice and blend until thick like ice cream.

> ## Frankie's Tip:
> This recipe has many variations; add CocoPro, unsweetened chocolate, coconuts or a frozen banana instead of the ice.

Phase 3 Desserts and Treats

Apple Cake

2 apples, peeled, cored
  and cut up
2 tbsp orange juice
1 cup almond butter
¼ cup Oh Agave
2 organic eggs

1 tbsp vanilla extract
2 tbsp cinnamon
½ tsp sea salt
1 cup unsweetened coconut
  (optional)
Coconut or olive oil spray

Preheat oven to 350°F. In a food processor combine the apple, orange juice. Pulse until well blended. Pulse in almond butter, agave, eggs, cinnamon and salt. Spray a small baking dish with either coconut oil or olive oil spray. Pour in mixture, sprinkle with unsweetened coconut (optional) and bake for 35-40 minutes.

**Gluten-Free/Sugar-Free
Apple Crisp**

6 Organic apples, peeled and
  cut up
1 tbsp lemon juice
1 tbsp vanilla extract
1 tbsp cinnamon

3 tbsp arrowroot powder
1½ cups of almond flour
¼ cup grape seed oil
¼ tsp sea salt
¼ cup organic coconut oil
¼ cup Oh Agave
Coconut or olive oil spray

Preheat oven to 350°F. Place apple slices in a large bowl, sprinkle with lemon juice, cinnamon, vanilla and arrowroot. Toss to coat the apples. In a small bowl combine almond flour, salt, coconut oil, grape seed oil and agave for the topping. Spray a 3 quart baking dish with either coconut or olive oil spray. Spread the apple mixture in the baking dish and crumble the topping over the apples. Cover and bake for 45 minutes until the apples are bubbling. Uncover and bake for 5-10 minutes. Serve warm or cold.

Frankie's Tip:

Whenever a recipe calls for oil, I use Barlean's organic coconut oil. It is considered to be a medium chain triglyceride and has many health benefits including being thermogenic. You will burn more calories while using it – awesome!

Phase 3 Desserts and Treats

Quick Apple Crunch
4-6 apples, peeled, cored
 and cut up
1 cup frozen berries, any kind
 (optional)
1 cup almond flour
½ cup assorted nuts, walnuts,
 almonds, pecans etc.
½ cup raisins
1 tsp vanilla
¼ cup butter
¼ cup coconut oil
½ cup palm sugar
 (looks like brown sugar),
 or Xylitol or Oh Agave
1 tbsp lemon juice
Coconut or olive oil spray

Preheat the oven to 350°F. Spray a baking dish with either the coconut or olive oil. Place the apples in the baking dish. In a small bowl, combine all of the other ingredients and spread on top of apples. Bake for 35 minutes. Take the cover off for the last 5-10 minutes making sure the raisins do not burn.

Frankie's Tip:
You can use both butter and coconut oil or either. This dish is great when you have company coming and want a quick wow dessert. The recipe is very forgiving and adaptable.

Double Chocolate Walnut Brownies
½ cup sugar free dark chocolate
 chips for batter
⅓ cup sugar free dark chocolate
 chips for topping
¼ cup coconut flour
¼ tsp sea salt
½ tsp baking soda
2 eggs
¼ cup Oh Agave nectar or
 palm sugar
¼ cup grape seed oil or
 coconut oil
1 tbsp vanilla extract
¼ cup chopped walnuts or
 macadamia nuts
Olive oil or coconut oil spray

Preheat oven to 350°F. Place ½ cup chocolate chips into a food processor and pulse to the consistency of coarse sand. Pulse in the coconut flour, salt and baking soda until combined. Pulse in eggs, agave, grape seed oil and vanilla. Grease an 8x8 Pyrex glass dish with the oil spray. Pour in batter and sprinkle walnuts and remaining chocolate chips over the top. Bake 25-30 minutes. Cool and serve.

Phase 3 Desserts and Treats

Bon Bons
4 large scoops whey powder
(we used unsweetened vanilla whey)
1 16 oz jar almond butter
1 tbsp salt

1 tbsp vanilla flavoring
¼ cup ground salba
Powdered Xylitol to taste
   (maybe ⅓ cup)
Chocolate candy, nuts, coconut

Mix together and put in fridge until firm. Then roll into balls. Dip in chocolate candy and then nuts and/or unsweetened coconut.

Chocolate Sauce
8 oz unsweetened baker's
   chocolate
1 dropper full vanilla Stevia

Powdered Xylitol to taste
Add coconut oil to thin
   (and cause it's so good for you!)

Cheesecake
3 8 oz packs of organic
   cream cheese
1 tsp of organic vanilla
1¼ cups of powdered Xylitol
(the original recipe calls for 1¾)
preferably, powderized in a
Vit-a-mix

1 cup of organic heavy cream
4 organic eggs
2 cups of organic sour cream
   (= one 1 lb container)
1 tbsp of lemon juice

Mix in the Vit-a-mix, or you can combine as follows: Beat the cream cheese first then gradually beat in the powdered Xylitol until very fluffy. Add eggs one at a time.....beating after each addition. Beat remaining ingredients, pour into crust and bake at 350°F for 1½ hours. Place pizza pan on bottom rack or directly under the cake to catch drippings.

Turn oven off and open oven a little. Let cake cool down in the oven. Keep in refrigerator.

Phase 3 Desserts and Treats

Chocolate Pudding

3 extra large eggs

½ cup of powdered organic
   dark chocolate (sugarless)

½ cup of Xylitol

1 tsp vanilla

½ cup of almond milk, soy
   creamer or any milk or
   non milk liquid product

¼ cup coconut oil or butter

Put all the ingredients in a sauce pan on low to medium heat and stir constantly until it thickens like custard. Remove from heat and pour into either a pie plate with almond flour and a little coconut oil and bake for a few minutes, or into ramekins. Put in the refrigerator and cool.

Frozen Cappuccino

1 cup crushed ice

5 drops of toffee Stevia

5 drops of chocolate Stevia

1 cup of coffee

Mix in blender until smooth. Pour into glass and serve.

Pumpkin Pie

1 15 oz can pumpkin

¾ tsp ground cinnamon

½ tsp ground nutmeg

¼ tsp ground ginger

¼ tsp ground cloves

½ tsp sea salt

1 ¼ cups cream

2 eggs, slightly beaten

About ⅓ cup powdered Xylitol
   (or add more if desired)

Mix pumpkin and spices together. Add remaining ingredients. Mix slowly just until thoroughly melted. Pour into pie shell (We used the cookie like pie crust, page 178 (make at least double the recipe, and we also added walnuts and cinnamon.) Bake at 425°F for 15 minutes, then reduce temperature to 350°F for an additional 30-40 minutes. Thoroughly cool pie before serving. Serves 6-8.

Coconut Flour Recipes

Make sure all ingredients are at room temperature for best results. When using coconut oil, it should be melted but not hot.

Banana Cake
½ cup butter, melted
½ cup coconut milk
12 eggs
1 tsp vanilla
1 cup powdered Xylitol
1 tsp salt
1½ tsp ground cinnamon

1 tsp ground nutmeg
½ tsp ground cloves
1 cup sifted coconut flour
1 tsp baking powder
2 cups grated zucchini
½ cup nuts, chopped
1 tsp banana flavoring

Combine butter, coconut milk, eggs, and vanilla. In a separate bowl mix together sugar, salt, and spices; stir into wet mixture. Combine coconut flour with baking powder and whisk into batter until there are no more lumps. Fold in zucchini and nuts. Pour batter into 2 greased 8-9 inch layer pans or one 9x9x2 pan. Bake at 350°F for approx. 40 minutes. Cool.

Coconut Bread
¾ cup sifted organic
   coconut flour
½ cup organic virgin
   coconut oil or butter, melted

6 eggs
2 tbsp Xylitol
½ tsp salt
1 tsp baking powder

Blend together eggs, butter, Xylitol and salt. Combine coconut flour with baking powder and whisk thoroughly into batter until there are no lumps. Pour into greased 9x5x3 inch or smaller loaf pan and bake at 350°F for 40 minutes. Remove from pan and cool on rack.

Coconut Flour Recipes

Coconut Flour Chocolate Cake
½ cup coconut oil
¼ cup cocoa powder
¼ cup coconut milk
9 eggs

1 ½ cups Xylitol
¾ tsp Himalayan salt
1 tsp vanilla extract
¾ cup sifted coconut flour
¾ tsp baking powder

Melt coconut oil in a saucepan over low heat or place jar in pan of warm water (note coconut oil easily melts and will congeal as it cools). Add cocoa powder and coconut milk and mix together. Remove from heat and set aside. In a bowl, mix together eggs, Xylitol, salt, and vanilla. Stir in cocoa mixture. Combine coconut flour with baking powder and whisk into batter until there are no lumps. Pour batter into greased 8x8x2 or 9x9x2-inch pan. Bake at 350°F for 35 minutes or until knife inserted into center comes out clean.

Salba (Chia) Banana Coconut Muffins
Combining the mild flavors of banana and coconut, these muffins are truly a unique healthy snack that your kids will love. Add raisins, cranberries, or blueberries to add a new dimension of texture.

2 tbsp coconut oil
3 room-temperature eggs
⅓ cup mashed banana
  (1 small, ripe banana)
1 tsp alcohol-free vanilla flavor
  or vanilla extract
¼ tsp salt

2 tbsp Salba whole seeds
¼ tsp baking powder
½ tsp ground cinnamon
1 tbsp shredded coconut
2 tbsp raisins, cranberries or
  blueberries (optional)
¼ cup coconut flour

Preheat oven to 400°F. Mix together oil, eggs, banana, vanilla, and salt. Add coconut flour, Salba, baking powder, cinnamon, and shredded coconut, and whisk together until smooth. Fold in raisins. Other options include dried cranberries, blueberries, walnuts, cashews or cacao nibs. Pour into muffin cups greased with coconut oil. Bake 15 minutes or until toothpick inserted in center of muffins comes out clean. Cool on wire rack. Makes 6 muffins.

Coconut Flour Recipes

Cookie-like Crust -
(Pastry Crust)
Crushed walnuts
3 tbsp coconut flour
1 tbsp almond or hazelnut flour
Melted butter (to bind)
1 egg

Bake 10 minutes at 350°F

Stevia (if desired)

(Should be dough like)
(Put walnuts with powdered
Xylitol to make Russian
Tea Cookies)

Sweet Nut Crust
(Can be used for Cheesecake)
1 cup roasted salted almonds
1 egg
4 tbsp coconut flour
2 tbsp almond flour

⅓ cup butter
About ¼ cup powdered
   Xylitol
1 package Stevia
Cinnamon

Pulse/Mix in blender. Press in the bottom of a glass pan. Bake at 225°F for
about 10 minutes.

Pancakes
2 eggs
2 tbsp organic virgin coconut
   oil or butter, melted
2 tbsp coconut milk or
   whole milk

1 tsp Xylitol
¼ tsp salt
2 tbsp sifted organic
   coconut Flour
¼ tsp baking powder

Blend together eggs, oil, coconut milk, sugar and salt. Combine coconut flour
with baking powder and thoroughly mix into batter. Heat 1 tbsp of coconut
oil in a skillet. Spoon batter onto hot skillet making pancakes about 2 to 3
inches in diameter. Batter will be thick, but will flatten out when cooking.
Makes about 8 pancakes.

Coconut Flour Recipes

Popovers
4 eggs
½ cup coconut milk

¼ tsp salt
2 tbsp sifted coconut flour
3 tbsp corn starch

With blender or whisk, blend together all ingredients until there are no lumps and batter is slightly bubbly. Fill greased muffin cups 2/3 full. Bake at 400°F for 20 minutes without opening oven door. Popovers will expand while cooking until they almost seem to pop over sideways. Makes 6 popovers. The popovers are best when served hot, immediately after removing from the oven.

Phase 3 Holiday Table

Here are some great ideas to use for a special occasion feast!

Vegetables

Oven Roasted Broccoli
1 bunch of broccoli

2 tbsp olive oil, coconut oil
or macadamia oil
½ tsp sea salt

Preheat the oven to 400°F. Wash and cut the broccoli into small pieces with long stems. In a large bowl, toss the broccoli with the oil and salt. Spread the broccoli on a baking sheet lines with parchment paper. Bake for 12-15 minutes until tender and slightly browned.

Grilled Portobello Mushrooms
3 large Portobello mushrooms

2 tbsp olive oil
1 tsp sea salt

Clean mushrooms and cut off stems. Rub mushrooms with olive oil and sprinkle with sea salt. Grill or broil for 4-5 minutes on each side.

Vegetables

Frankie's Butternut Squash

1 butternut squash, peeled and
   cut up (I use the pre cut pkg.)
¼ cup orange juice

1 tsp vanilla
1 tbsp Oh Agave
1 tbsp butter or coconut oil
Olive oil or coconut oil spray

Preheat the oven to 350°F. Grease a baking dish with the oil spray. Cover and bake for 25 minutes until soft. In a large bowl, mash the squash and incorporate the rest of the ingredients. Serve.

Mashed Cauliflower

2 heads of cauliflower, washed
   and cut into large pieces

2 tbsp organic butter or
   coconut oil or 1 tbsp each
½ tsp sea salt

Preheat oven to 350°F. Steam cauliflower until very tender. Either puree cauliflower in a food processor or mash with a fork. Mix in butter and/or coconut oil and salt. Bake in a casserole dish for 20 minutes. Serve warm.

Frankie's Tip:
Sauté onions and mushrooms and season with salt and pepper.

Desserts

**Pumpkin Cinnamon
Cheesecake**

1 medium pie pumpkin, acorn
   squash or butternut squash
1 quart whole milk yogurt
   strained overnight up to
   24 hours, discard whey

½ cup Oh Agave nectar,
   palm sugar or Xylitol
1 tbsp vanilla extract
1 tbsp lemon juice
1 tbsp cinnamon
¼ tsp sea salt
Olive oil or coconut oil spray

Preheat oven to 350°F. Fill the bottom of a baking dish with ¼ inch of water. Cut pumpkin in half, remove seeds and place face down in baking dish. Roast for 45-55 minutes until soft. Allow pumpkin to cool and scrape flesh into a bowl. In a food processor, combine 2 cups of pumpkin, the strained yogurt, Oh Agave, vanilla and lemon juice. Process until smooth 1-2 minutes. Process in cinnamon and salt. Grease a 9 inch tart pan with the oil spray and pour in batter. Bake 45-50 minutes, until firm. Cool and serve.

Desserts

Open Apple Pie
6-8 apples, peeled, cored
   and cut up
1 tbsp lemon juice
1 cup almond flour for crust
1 tbsp almond flour for the pie
¼ cup butter or coconut oil
1 tbsp cinnamon

1 ½ tsp vanilla
¼ cup raisins
¼ cup walnuts or pecans
¼ cup Xylitol, palm sugar
   (coconut sugar, low glycemic)
   or Oh Agave
¼ tsp arrow root
Olive oil or coconut oil spray

Preheat the oven to 350°F. Grease a pie plate with the oil spray. In a bowl, mix the almond flour and butter or coconut oil. Press the mixture onto the pie plate making a bottom crust. Bake for 5-6 minutes. In a bowl, combine all of the other ingredients and toss with the cut up apple. Pour into the pie plate and bake for 30-35 minutes.

Lemon Tart
Crust:
1 tbsp coconut oil or butter
1 cup almond flour for crust

Tart:
¾ cup fresh lemon juice
1 tsp lemon oil extract
   (optional)
¾ cup Xylitol or palm sugar
4 eggs
2 egg yolks

Preheat oven to 350°F. Grease a pie plate with the oil spray. In a bowl, mix the almond flour and butter or coconut oil. Press the mixture onto the pie plate making a bottom crust. Bake for 5-6 minutes. In a saucepan over medium heat, whisk together the lemon juice, lemon juice extract, Xylitol, eggs and egg yolks constantly whisking until the filling looks like pudding. Pour onto crust and refrigerate until serving.

Frankie's Tip:
This can be made with or without the crust. I sometimes beat eggs whites for the top and place under the broiler to brown to make it into a lemon meringue pie. No cream of tartar in the egg whites, please. It is loaded with gluten.

Desserts

Gluten-Free & Vegan
Peppermint Patties
¼ cup coconut oil
¼ cup Oh Agave

½ tsp peppermint oil,
  organic preferred
½ -1 cup sugar free dark
  chocolate chips, melted

In a small bowl, combine coconut oil, agave and peppermint oil. Mash any clumps of coconut oil until the mixture is smooth. Freeze mixture for 5 minutes until it starts to harden. Line a plate with parchment paper. Using a 1½ tsp ice cream scoop, measure out little balls and place on the plate. Put the plate in the freezer and freeze until firm. Remove from freezer, leaving the balls on the parchment, flatten into little patties. Using a spoon, dip patties into melted chocolate and put back on parchment lined plate to harden for 10 minutes. During warm summer months you may have to refreeze.

Gluten-Free Coconut
Macaroons
6 organic egg whites
¼ tsp sea salt

½ cup Oh Agave
1 tbsp vanilla extract
3 cups unsweetened shredded
  coconut

Preheat oven to 350°F. In a mixing bowl, whisk egg whites and salt until stiff. Fold in agave, vanilla and coconut. Line a baking sheet with parchment paper. Drop batter onto parchment paper, one rounded tablespoon at a time (aprox. 12). Pinch each one (like a kiss). Bake for 10-15 minutes. Serve.

Frankie's Tip:
I like to dip these in melted sugar-free dark chocolate.

Endnotes

1. Liang, Lan, PhD, et al., "Will All Americans Become Overweight or Obese? Estimating the Progression and Cost of the US Obesity Epidemic," Obesity 2008 Jul 24;16(10):2323-30

2. Whitaker RC, Wright JA, Pepe MS, Seidel KD, Dietz WH. Predicting obesity in young adulthood from childhood and parental obesity. *N Engl J Med* 1997; 37(13):869–873.

3. Wang, Youfa and May A. Beydoun, "The Obesity Epidemic in the United States," Epidemiologic Reviews, doi:10.1093/epirev/mxm007 ibid.

4. Devlin, Kate, "One in 10 children in England 'will be obese within five years'," The Telegraph, UK, 15 December 2009, http://tinyurl.com/yj2x5pu

5. New Zealand Ministry of Health, "Obesity in New Zealand," http://www.moh.govt.nz/obesity

6. www.mcph.org

7. http://edoc.unibas.ch/531/1/DissB_7757.pd7

8. World Health Organization, "Obesity and Overweight," 2003, retrieved 27 April 2009 IBID

9. CDC, "Study Estimates Medical Cost of Obesity May Be As High As $147 Billion Annually," 27 July 2009, http://www.cdc.gov/media/pressrel/2009/r090727.htm

10. Colagiuri, S. et al., "The cost of overweight and obesity in Australia," Medical J. Australia 2010 Mar 1; 192(5):260-64

11. Schacht, Henry, "Slim Pickings: Buy Weight Watchers International Inc.," GuruFocus.com, 18 January 2010, http://www.gurufocus.com/news.php?id=81900

12. Morales, T., "Gastric Bypass Surgery Gone Bad," CBSNews.com, 21 January 2005, http://tinyurl.com/5ckrp

13. Simeons, A.T.W., Pounds and Inches: A new approach to obesity, Rome, 1976 (privately published); available at http://hcgdietinfo.com/hCG_Diet-Dr.-Simeons-Manuscript.htm

14. Becker, Robert O., MD, and Gary Selden, The Body Electric: Electromagnetism and the Foundation of Life, William Morrow, 1985, pp. 284-85

15. Lai, Henry, Dr., "Mobile Phones: Is there a Health Risk?," paper presented at the IBC-UK Conference, 16–17 September 1997, in Brussels, Belgium; at http://www.mapcruzin.com/radiofrequency/henry_lai1.htm .

16. Belluscio, Daniel Oscar, MD, http://www.oralhcg.com/english/in7.htm#1

17. Simeons, A.T.W., "The action of chorionic gonadotropin in the obese," The Lancet 1954 Nov 6; 267(6845):946-947

18. Belluscio, Daniel Oscar, MD, "Utility of an Oral Presentation of hCG (Human Chorionic Gonadotrophin) for the Management of Obesity: A Double-blind Study," at http://www.hcgobesity.org/international_workshop/welcome_frm.htm

19. Human chorionic gonadotropin (hCG) prevents the transformed phenotypes induced by 17 estradiol in human breast epithelial cells Hilal Kocdor[a], Mehmet A. Kocdor[a], Jose Russo[a], Kara E. Snider[a], Johana E. Vanegas[a], Irma H. Russo[a] and Sandra V. Fernandez[,a,] Fox Chase Cancer Center, Breast Cancer Research Laboratory, 333 July 2009.

20. Treatment with human chorionic gonadotropin and risk of breast cancer. L Bernstein, R Hanisch, J Sullivan-Halley and R K Ross Cancer Epidemiol Biomarkers Prev July 1995 4; 437

21. Journal of Clinical Oncology, 2006 ASCO Annual Meeting Proceedings (Post-Meeting Edition). Vol 24, No 18S (June 20 Supplement), 2006: 10658 © 2006 American Society of Clinical OncologyHuman chorionic gonadotropin (hCG) induction of apoptosis in breast cancer W. B. Carter and M. Sekharam

22. Dayami Lopez, Madhavi Sekharam, Domenico Coppola and W. Bradford Carter Don and Erika Wallace. Comprehensive Breast Program, H. Lee Moffitt Cancer Center and Research Institute, Tampa, Florida

23. Human Chorionic Gonadotropin Decreases Proliferation and Invasion of Breast Cancer MCF-7 Cells by Inhibiting NF-B and AP-1 Activation* Ch. V. Rao, X. Li, S. K. Manna, Z. M. Lei, and B. B. Aggarwal J. Biol. Chem., Vol. 279, Issue 24, 25503-25510, June 11, 2004

24. Human chorionic gonadotropin (hCG) and prevention of breast cancer Jaak Ph. Janssens[a], José Russo[d], Irma Russo[d], Luc Michiels[a], Gilbert Donders[b], Marcel Verjans[b], Ine Riphagen[b], Thierry Van den Bossche[b], Marijke Deleu[b] and Peter Sieprath[c] [a]University of Hasselt, Hasselt, Belgium [b]H. Hart Hospital, Tienen, Belgium [c]Ziekenhuis Oost-Limburg, Genk, Belgium [d]The Fox Chase Cancer Centre, Philadelphia, USA

25. *Direct hCG Actions Afford Protection Against Breast Cancer.* Irma H. Russo, Jose RussoBreast Cancer Research Laboratory, Fox Chase Cancer Center, Philadelphia, PA, USA

Resources

Dr. Simeons' book, *Pounds and Inches,* is freely available on many websites.

Recommended hCG Resources

Anumed-International 888.921.3880

Anumed-International offers the most potent effective, highly energized Homeopathic hCG.

E-hCG has additional Amino Acids to increase mental clarity, glucose conversion and additional fat releasing. Experience increased energy, fat-burning and body sculpting from those "hard to lose" places. Anumed-Intl. also offers a Vitamin D3 cream that is 10,000 IU per pump and a perfect supplement to add to your e-hCG diet!

E-Mail: care@anumed-intl.com
Website: www.Anumed-Intl.com

Stevia International 888.921.3880

Stevia is the perfect addition to your e-hCG Diet! Stevia is an herb that is sweeter than sugar but is calorie free and does not spike your blood sugar and is even safe for diabetics. Stevia International offers a wide variety of liquid and powder Stevia products: Natural, Vanilla, Toffee, Mango, Peach, Pomegranate and many more.

E-Mail: care@stevia-intl.com
Website: www.Stevia-Intl.com

About the Author

Sherrill Sellman, N.D., Naturopathic Doctor (Board Certified in Integrative Medicine), is an educator, women's natural health expert, psychotherapist and journalist in the field of women's health. She is also, a much sought after international lecturer, host of two weekly radio shows, senior editor and contributing writer to numerous health publications. Dr. Sellman is the best- 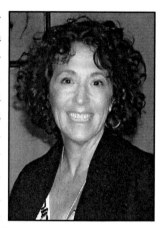 selling author of *Hormone Heresy: What Women MUST Know*, *What Women MUST Know to Protect Their Daughters from Breast Cancer* and *The Return of the Ancient Seed*. Her professional credentials and commitment to an integrative healing approach extends over a 30-year period.

www.whatwomenmustknow.com
www.myultimatefatloss.com

About the Co-Author

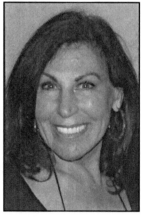

Frankie Boyer, an impassioned voice for holistic living, has attracted tens of thousands of guests on her award-winning holistic health and lifestyle radio shows. Her shows focus on a diverse and broad range of topics from timely male and female issues to longevity and health, spirituality, and the environment, to money, movies and celebrity news. Frankie Boyer is a powerful voice for everyone searching for useful insights and information on traditional and alternative approaches to lifestyle, health care and well being. She spreads sound advice from experts—to educate listeners on how to take personal responsibility for their own health and graceful aging. Frankie is a passionate cook, creating nutrient dense, low-carb, gluten-free, sugar-free and vegetarian recipes. She specializes in hCG recipes.

www.frankieboyer.com

For other titles
or a free catalog
call 800-729-4131
or visit www.nohoax.com